Starving for Affection

a journey of eating disorders, drugs, and sex

by

Nancy Lee Bausch, Ph.D

iUniverse, Inc.
New York   Bloomington

Starving for Affection
a journey of eating disorders, drugs, and sex

iUniverse books may be ordered through booksellers or by contacting:

*iUniverse
1663 Liberty Drive
Bloomington, IN 47403
www.iuniverse.com
1-800-Authors (1-800-288-4677)*

*ISBN: 978-1-4401-1151-8 (sc)
ISBN: 978-1-4401-1152-5 (ebook)*

Printed in the United States of America

iUniverse rev. date: 1/30/2009

Chapter 1

"Mother, May I?"

Sometimes you have to look back so you can move forward. None of us wants to be an addict. That's not the wish little girls make before they blow out their birthday candles. I didn't have to worry about the cake and the candles, though, after I turned twelve.

Mother seldom baked for us. She didn't feel she had to. Not like her job where she had to make everyone love her. So it was only on those special occasions that we would get the benefit of her baking expertise in the kitchen. At her work, every day was a special occasion. Cakes, pies, cookies, and candy flooded the premises where it was vital that she get her daily doses of what she needed – their gratitude, appreciation, and unending affection.

In our house, we knew the grandparents were coming to visit and it was my father's birthday if there was the glorious sight of a fresh-baked cake resting in a shiny gray container on the Formica kitchen counter.

My younger sister's birthdays were held at places where they held parties. Her roster of friends was growing year by year. Our house couldn't hold all her giggling, cherubic girlfriends eager to come to her birthday parties. My father had always had birthday cake when he was a kid. Mother grudgingly supplied him with the requisite cake every year, especially when the grandparents made it their yearly visit to our home.

After the age of twelve, Mother didn't make birthday cakes for me. She said she didn't want to encourage my weight gain, so it was better not to have temptation in the house. I would get money to go to the movies. Mother had checked to see what a child's ticket would cost. But I couldn't get in on a child's ticket anymore. Even though technically I wouldn't be an adult for several years, I was always challenged about my age due to how large I was.

"That'll be five dollars." The cashier had looked up briefly from the book she was reading.

"I need a child's ticket. I'm twelve." I would respond hopefully, as the line of people behind me was growing larger.

"You're too big for twelve. Do you have I.D.?" What did she expect me to have to show her I was not an adult? Not too many twelve-year-olds carry their birth certificates to the movies with them. I could hear irritated murmurs behind me.

"We're gonna miss the previews. What's the problem?"

"Looks like some teenager tryin' to buy a kid's ticket for herself."

Heads turned to look. Desiccated turtle-necked men and women slowly leaned their way around the people in front of them.

"I'm really only twelve. I just have enough for a child's ticket," I pleaded as quietly as possible. Maybe she would take pity on me.

Yeah, sure.

2

Mad that I was keeping her from her romance novel, she spoke loudly through the hole in the glass.

"I'll get the manager. You can talk to him."

The crowd was getting more than restless.

"Now what?"

"They're getting the manager."

"Jesus Christ, I won't have time to get any popcorn before the movie starts."

My face bright red from embarrassment, I quickly glanced around to reassure the last voice that I would be done in just a minute.

When I saw the swollen body and blotched face of a woman who had spent too many hours at the snack bar, I sighed and moved away from the ticket booth.

I went instead to a store, used the ticket money for as many chocolate bars as I could get, and then walked a mile to the closest mall, eating all the way.

When I got to the pet store, I spent most of the movie time looking at the puppies playing behind the squared glass enclosures. As I moved from one to the other, I sang under my breath, "Happy birthday to me, happy birthday to me."

After that, I didn't even try to get into the movies. As usual for my next couple of birthdays, Mother would drop me off with enough money for a child's ticket. I knew I couldn't ask for more money because they thought I was an adult. I could hear the likely recriminations coming from her in my head.

"Mother, could I have a little more money?"

"Why do you need more? That's the exact amount you need. I checked to make sure." I would get a suspicious glance.

"Are you trying to get more to buy snacks? You know how we feel about that." I assumed the "we" was my father since I had never been consulted.

"No, I wouldn't do that. It's just that they think I'm an adult."

"What! Did you see any of my friends there or any of the neighbors?"

Nope. This wasn't a conversation I wanted to have with my mother.

So I would wait until she had turned the corner, make my way to the nearest candy store to buy my emotional binge food and then head to the mall.

Right down memory lane I stumble, my mother nipping at the edges of my mind, like the Alpha shark getting ready to explode in an eating frenzy.

This day was my father's birthday. Mother had baked a cake. She wasn't in a good mood.

"What have you done now?" I knew I was in for it when she glared at me over the desecrated cake tins.

"Couldn't you wait two hours, for God's sake?" She disgustedly slammed the frosting bowl in front of me on the kitchen counter.

"And don't eat any of that frosting. I don't have time to make more. You'll need every bit of it to fill in those holes you made in the cake layers."

"But Mother, I didn't..." I began to feebly protest.

She interrupted, "We have your grandparents coming in an hour. They give me a hard time, anyway, about your weight."

She sighed as she put the two cake layers on a serving plate. I dreaded that sigh. It had all the "woe is me" of the world in it. I heard that sigh at least twenty times a day.

"Mom, I haven't been in here at all. I've been up in my room getting ready."

She had hollered for me to come down to the kitchen. I should have known from the irritation in her voice that I had somehow upset her. I had run down the stairs as fast as I could. I knew it would be worse if I kept her waiting. I knew my face was flushed from the exertion. And I had put on the horrible instrument of female torture she had laid on my bed that morning. I had to pull it up as far as I could on the upper half of my body to corral as much of the excess flesh as I could. Then I'd have to breathe carefully or my chest would puff out and the reinforced elastic top of the girdle would start noisily rolling down my body like curling tar on a hot road. Unfortunately, the blood being pushed up in place of the air had bubbled up to my face. Maybe she thought I looked guilty when she saw my red cheeks and the sweat running from my hairline to my neck. It didn't help that I had to keep swiping at it so it wouldn't drip down in front of her.

"That reminds me. Did you put on the new girdle I got you at the Plus Women's store yesterday? Your other one was all stretched out."

She had turned her back on me and was knifing along the edge of the circular pans resting on the long, sand-colored kitchen counter.

"Yes, Mother. It sure feels tight, though. Could I maybe wear one of my long sweaters instead?"

"For Christ's sake, of course it's tight. That's not the girdle's fault. And no, it's August. Your grandmother would know right away you were trying to hide your body with a hot sweater in the summer. Don't you have any sense at all?"

I knew that was a rhetorical question since she always knew the answer. I just waited as usual, my hands busy trying to keep the perspiration from falling into the oversized bowl of pink icing. My father's cake always had pink icing. Mother liked pink icing since it made her cakes stand out at work. She had a ready supply of the ingredients to make pink icing. I don't know if my father ever complained about the color. I think he was just happy that he got a cake.

God, I hated anything pink. It told me I wasn't the Barbie-doll size of the other little girls whose mothers never had to worry about buying feminine garments to hold in their kid's stomach, thighs, and butt. Mother had finally given up on finding anything to fit me in the Girls' section of the clothing store. She would gaze sadly at the rows of cute little pink tops and abbreviated shorts the popular girls at school wore as she dragged me to the Women's side of the store to sort through the racks looking for something she called "at least presentable" for me to appear in. I think she was more worried about how I looked when I was with her than what I needed for school clothes.

When she had to go shopping with me, she often asked for oversized bags for the saleswoman to put the purchased items in at the clothes stores that catered to large women. Then she'd tell me to put the oversized plastic bags in front of me as we walked through the mall back to the car. I think she wanted to minimize me as much as she could with whatever she could find when we infrequently went out together. I don't remember her taking me someplace that was not on the agenda for getting me ready to go back into the world of school.

"Stand sideways so you look thinner," she'd whisper frantically to me when by some misfortune we'd run into one of her friends from work or the neighborhood. It was more embarrassing and humiliating than usual for my mother if they had their normal-sized daughters with them and Mother would have to compare me to theirs. She would try to get in front of me, pushing me back with her hands behind her as I tried to get into a position that didn't look like I weighed as much as I did.

"It's so nice to see you. Is that your beautiful daughter with you? My, she looks like a model!" Mother gushed as she bunched her hands into fists behind her back.

When I saw those fingers begin to curl, I tried to back up, but I was never far enough back for her not to reach me. Somehow she could sense I was moving like a wart hog trying to escape in a river of piranhas. She seemed to move faster than the speed of light as she punched me in the stomach without missing a beat in her one-way conversation with whoever I was embarrassing her this particular time.

"Well, it sure is wonderful to chat with you. We don't get too much time at work to just talk, do we?" She was taking paces back as she didn't wait for the woman and her daughter to respond. With a last sickly grin, like a chimpanzee trained with a cattle prod to show its teeth for the movie camera, she'd turn away, still keeping me from anyone's view.

She'd turn me around so fast I often got dizzy and had to hold onto her to regain my balance.

"Don't you dare faint. C'mon, we have to get further away. They're still watching us."

She grabbed my hand clutching her and yanked me along next to her as she rapidly made her way to the store's exit. I would be holding the oversized bags, which were now bumping against our legs as she pulled me towards the exit doors.

"Mother, could you…"

"Don't even think about stopping. Oh, that was so humiliating. What will I say to her at work about you? Maybe she didn't see the bags with the store's name on them. Damn it all to hell."

The scenario really didn't change much if we were caught by someone she knew when we were on a shopping trip. When I'd hear her cuss under her breath as we came out of a store, I'd know we'd go through this awful social ritual.

After one of those unforeseen meetings at the mall, I'd come home, slink up the stairs with the bags loaded with unattractive women's wear. The clothes were heavy since more material was needed to make them for teenage tubbies. But I didn't feel the plastic loops cutting into my forearms. I just needed to escape from my mother as soon as I could or she would take another opportunity to lengthily tear me down.

On those many occasions I couldn't move fast enough to make it up the stairs halfway to my sanctuary/bedroom so I could say I couldn't hear her calling me back, she'd make me stand in front of her while she berated me for my appearance. The big plastic bags would start to saw into my flesh. It was almost as if she knew even the clothing containers didn't like me either.

She didn't try to hide her frustration and contempt. I had made her look bad in front of others. It didn't matter that she probably didn't like them anyway. It reflected on her that I was a walking twelve-year-old tub of lard.

Hands on her hips, she'd regard me with a baleful stare and start in: "Of all people to run into, it had to be that snippy secretary and her little snob of a daughter. And right in front of the Plus Women's store. I could tell what she was thinking. That fake smile. Her daughter looking bored. They couldn't wait to get away from us. I know I'll hear about it at work. All the ladies will know I have to shop in the fat stores for you."

She paused while she actually contemplated what she would say to them at work. Not looking at me but off in the distance, her eyes narrowed and her mouth pursed: "I'll tell them you had a growth spurt. All girls at puberty still have some baby fat. I'll let slip that you're big boned like your father."

Thinking I had a chance to make an end run around her to get away, I'd start to move. Her snake sensor would kick in. She'd sense her victim was getting loose, so even though she wasn't looking directly at me, she shifted her body to block the attempt.

"I'm not through with you yet. Don't even think of going up those stairs until I'm done," she would hiss.

I had seen a news story once about a cow that had bolted from the truck taking it to the slaughterhouse. It had remained free for several days. As the reporter began telling about the escapade, I felt myself rooting for that lone creature trying to avoid its death. Maybe it got away. Somebody would help it. A family would call the station to say they would adopt it. It was not to be. The last live shot showed the captured emaciated cow in the back of a wood-slated truck. It was looking over its shoulder. All the fear and pain shown in its expression as it sought the camera. Perhaps she thought her pleading eyes would give her a chance to survive.

As I remembered the story while Mother was keeping me from freedom, I empathized with that poor cow again. In this instant, my eyes probably had the same look. Like her, I was recaptured, as Mother's arm became a bar across my chest.

"Why couldn't your sister have been with me when I ran into them? I could show her off. They would have been so jealous."

Even though I fought it, tears would start to slip from the corners of my eyes. I bent my head towards the carpet.

At that point, she'd turn back to me and scrutinize my figure. "How did you get like this? Your sister is so thin. I'm going to have to watch you like a hawk so you're not overeating."

She'd notice I had my head down.

"Look at me when I'm talking to you."

I'd raise my tear-stained face and murmur miserably, "I'm sorry."

"Well, you should be. Now I have to worry about going to work on Monday and seeing that woman." She turned her head in the direction of the kitchen.

"I know. I'll make some oatmeal raisin cookies for her. I'll say how low calorie they are. That way she'll think I don't cook fattening foods at home so it won't be my fault that you look like a house."

This scene repeated itself so many times I could have mouthed the words coming from her. They were never kind. I'd stand in front of her with that sad cow-eyed look, trapped and mute with grief.

Although nobody noticed, I never ate red meat after I had seen that doomed animal on TV. Maybe some cow somewhere would be given a second chance

"Hey, let's not send this one to the slaughterhouse. We'll keep her in memory of that girl who doesn't eat beef anymore because she wants us to save one."

Stupidly illogical, but I was twelve, and profit margin wasn't part of my vocabulary. Sometimes, I let my emotions rule my head. In my mind, some cow didn't die because I gave up eating them. Besides, I wanted to be a vet. I thought all vets never ate their prospective patients. It must be part of the veterinarian code: "Thou shalt not eat thy four-legged fellow creatures."

Anyway, if I was lucky, my skinny sister, who probably was the one who dug out pieces of the cooling birthday cake, would come racing in to tell Mother about her latest social success with the neighborhood pre-teens who gathered around her like she was Venus on the half shell. The fact that I made straight "As" was pretty low on the bragging scale for my mother. It was all about what people saw, and my younger sister was cute, loved pink, and was enthusiastically admired by all she encountered. Her framed school pictures marched complacently up the wall of our staircase, each one portending the wonderful future this attractive little princess would have.

I made sure I was definitely at home on School Photo Day. I didn't need a visual trail of my physical faults, even if my mother would have placed them next to my sister's. Now that I think of it, nobody ever asked where mine were as they gazed affectionately at the blossoming beauty of my sister carefully positioned each year in antique-white frames on the staircase wall.

I did forget once in elementary school to stay home when they took the yearly school photos. It was another unforgettable experience in the life of the unwanted.

It had been a sun-drenched morning at my elementary school. I was feeling good about the essay I had written about my future career as a veterinarian. Yep, you're right. Animals would love me unconditionally. And they couldn't make nasty comments about my looks. The ideal career for a fat female.

Our teacher, thin as a needle, of course, was just about to hand back the essays when the announcement came on:

"Teachers, would you please escort your classes to the gym for school pictures."

My face fell. The smile I had on because I just knew I was going to get that paper back with a bright red "A" dropped out of sight. I could feel my fingernails making furrows in my palms as my hands spasmodically curled into fists.

Oh no! I had forgotten to look at my calendar. I always circled the horrible School Picture Day so I could plan ahead to be sick, but I was only thinking about seeing that perfect essay handed back to me. I had concentrated on my fantasy of grinning proudly at the teacher and casually holding it in my hand flat so my envious classmates could see the big red-inked letter at the top.

I was panic-stricken. How was I going to get out of this?

"Teacher, could I please go to the bathroom?"

I could hide there until the lines of children passed by and then go to the School Nurse with a stomachache. I'd writhe a little and groan when she saw me. I could probably get a half an hour out of her, depending on my "sick kid" performance. She'd definitely keep me there for as long as it took for those awful pictures to be taken.

"Not now. We have to get to the gym right away."

She had the classroom door open and could see the other classes moving down the hallway.

I resigned myself to the fact that I had to have my picture taken. Maybe the photographer would do it fast. Like getting a shot in your arm when you weren't looking because the doctor was distracting you.

Of course not. The gods were against me - again. We were lined up next to this backdrop of some leaf-strewn yard in some part of the country that only existed in somebody's strange artistic imagination. Nothing like garish oranges and reds in fallen dead leaves to show off the cute kids. Didn't these people ever think of subdued colors so the person didn't jump right out of the picture at you?

Nope. It was a huge abnormally orange pumpkin for Thanksgiving; an enormous eight-foot green tree with big, flashing colored bulbs for Christmas, and humongous decorated eggs at Easter making the kid in the photo look like she had fallen down Alice's rabbit hole and ended up in a grotesque garden of frightening, neon plastic globes.

I guessed I wouldn't be fading into the background, as I craned my neck to get a look at the backdrop before we started to move forward.

So, it would be over in a minute, anyway. I'd be back in our classroom as quickly as it took to sit down on their little stool for a second, hear the click of the camera, and then the bellowed word "Next" as another kid took my place.

I would get my essay back and mentally drool over it while my classmates appeared jealous of the one attribute I didn't mind being oversized – my brain.

Wait a minute here. Just a second. Everyone can see the person get situated on the stool and the photographer coming over to tilt the chin up. Jeez, we're lined up behind the camera.

I wasn't overjoyed to realize all my peers who made fun of my women's clothes and my chipmunk cheeks were going to be an audience while I was getting my photo taken.

I watched as the photographer quickly positioned each person and placed the kid's face in the best position for the maximum benefit of the camera.

When several of the students in the class had finished, our teacher took them back to the classroom with instructions to us to return as soon as we were through.

I relaxed and patted my hair down as I waited my turn.

This is gonna be a breeze. He isn't taking long at all. I just won't look at their mean snotty little faces when I sit down.

I took the time now to check out everything involved in this photo process. As I glanced at the stool, the thought came into my head.

That stool is really small and it can move.

Not only did the three-legged stool look like it was built for a toddler, the thing had wheels on each of its legs.

"Okay, so just try not to move at all when you sit," I murmured when I noticed the stool size and the little black wheels.

The class bully leaned his bulbous head around his compatriots when he heard me.

"Try not to break it, Fatso, before we get our turn," he hollered from further back in the line. I could hear answering laughter as my face turned as red as overripe tomatoes, and my shoulders slumped in on themselves to try to make my front look as small as possible. I put my hands behind my back in an effort to cover my rear as much as I could, with my palms splayed out and facing the person behind me while I took a death grip on my wrists.

There were two in front of me. Both of them turned to see what was happening. I lowered my face and said, "I wonder when these'll be ready."

One of the two, a skanky-looking girl with acne like overflowing volcanoes, looked at me with haughty contempt. I guess I was the only person in the class who she could pick on with impunity. Even oozing acne sores were better than being fat.

"What do you care? The camera'll probably break anyway when you get in front of it." She sniffed and turned back to face the front so quickly some of the white pus from her face flew out and landed on her collar.

I'm gonna be sick, I thought to myself as I looked away from the splattered mess.

You can't upchuck now. That'll only make it worse. They'll not only be repulsed by the vomit, they'd comment on its size.

"Gross! Move back!"

"What happened?"

"That fat girl threw up!"

Their ugly scrunched faces would crinkle in disgust.

Some kid at the front of the line with me would yell back to the others.

"Oh man, that stinks. And it's all over the place."

"Yeah, well, she *is* fat. It's probably all the food she ate before she got here."

I mentally shivered as I imagined that dialogue. I shut my eyes and crept forward as I felt the skank move away from me.

When I opened them, I was staring at the garish backdrop. It was my turn.

I moved so fast towards the stool, I ran into it and pushed it into the backdrop.

Just what I need, I said bitterly to myself, as I made a grab for it before it rolled underneath the colored cloth, and I'd be left standing there with my face flush against that horrid picture.

The photographer was faster. He leaned down and caught one of its metal legs with one hand and stopped its momentum. He didn't look at me as he began to roll it back in front of the camera. I tried to sit on it as soon as it stopped rolling, but he still had one hand on the seat as he was pulling it. I was mortified. I had sat on his hand!

Oh my God, I can't believe this is happening.

I got up as fast as I could and looked at his hand.

"I'm really sorry. Is it okay?"

As the photographer shook it to get some feeling back into it, I could hear the guffaws from my peers as the next one in line told the one behind what had just happened. Word traveled down that line like spit off a mouthpiece knocked out in a boxing match. My father loved to watch the fights on television. Maybe it was cathartic for him since he never won any rounds with my mother.

Suddenly, instead of waiting in line, my remaining classmates had grouped themselves around the photo area.

I looked desperately at the photographer as he stationed himself next to the camera. He picked up the dangling cord connected to the camera with a small silver ring. I could see his thumb positioned over the red button he had to depress to take the picture.

Please, please, I prayed to myself, since obviously no heavenly intervention was going to save me, *don't come over here and move me around.*

I thought I was home free. He looked through the camera and started to push the button. He stopped in mid-thumb push.

God help me! I thought frantically to myself. Maybe God would take pity and get involved here.

Nope. As usual, my plea went unheeded. Maybe God was on a lunch break. He always seemed to be out of the office when I called. Wait. Could it be that God doesn't love fat girls, either?

As I pondered my switch to atheism, the photographer said, "Could you move a little to your left?"

I tried to shift my weight to my left. I couldn't move. It was like I was stuck to the plastic seat cover. I looked down at myself. Unthinkingly, I had made my legs go under the seat and behind the two back metal legs so I couldn't fall off. I would have to get them out one at a time, or I'd fall over with the stool attached and on top of me.

I frantically attempted to get my legs unstuck. The photographer was coming towards me to help.

"Do you need some help?"

"No, I can do it. Just give me a minute."

Meanwhile, the snickering in the bunch stationed around the photo area was getting louder. I could hear their comments as I tried to pull my legs out.

"Do you see that? She's stuck."

"How can you tell? I can't even see the stool!"

"Wait'll I tell Beth." "Beth" was in another class. The whole school would know by lunchtime.

I finally managed to get one leg out. It had a deep groove from being pushed so hard into the metal leg. I pulled my skirt down as far as I could on the side so they couldn't see the back of my leg. The other came free. I moved to the left.

"Now could you look to your right a little?" He was looking at the camera's framing shot. "Tilt your head back. Can you put your hair behind your ears?"

Oh sure, now everyone can see my double chin and the sides of my cheeks. **Is** *there no justice in this world?* I dramatically cried to myself.

"This'll be over in a minute," the photographer said as he pushed the button.

Maybe for you. For me, it won't be over ever.

I made my way through the throng of laughing kids who would continue to harass and humiliate me whenever they could get away with it.

Suddenly it seemed like my likely red "A" on the paper I would get back in a few minutes wasn't important, after all.

"Maybe the School Nurse has something for a headache," I said softly to myself as I headed for her office.

No, there weren't any proud pictures of me next to my sister on our family "Hall of Fame" wall. The certificate with the fifty gold stars for every book read had been pinned to the corkboard above my desk. I showed it to my father, hoping he would want to bring it to my mother's attention. Would this be the moment when I would get congratulated on something

I did? Would my father tell my mother how proud he was of me?

I had forgotten that he avoided my mother when he was in the house, just like now when she had me in her sights and was verbally flailing away.

I still had that gold-star-filled certificate of merit somewhere in my desk. I had removed it after Mother didn't notice it when she came into my room.

It had been a while since I had thought about that school picture day. I guess when my eyes focused on my sister's photos on the wall so I didn't have to look into my mother's disappointed and furious face, it all came back to me.

When the school pictures came back, I didn't look at them. I shoved a piece of paper in the front of the packet where the large picture would be. While my classmates were comparing theirs and cutting out the small ones to exchange, I put mine in my book bag.

That day I stopped at a fast-food restaurant on my way home and bought several of their biggest hamburgers, three bags of fries and the most gargantuan soda they had. I always saved the lunch money Mother put in a plastic see-through bag and placed in the front zippered pocket of my book bag. As she zipped it up, she would remind me not to buy anything fattening in the school cafeteria.

I had long ago stopped going into the school lunchroom. It was just another place where I would be taunted and embarrassed. I stayed in the classroom and read.

Now, as I finished eating every last bit of the greasy burgers and heavily salted French fries and washed them down with gulps of the soda at one of the fast-food places' outside tables, I scrunched up the white bags, poured out the ice from the drained soda cup and threw them away in the waste container built like a clown.

On top of the garbage, I stuffed in my school photo packet.

As I remembered the emotional eating binge I had done on that past day while Mother was still raving in my face now, I hoped my father would come home so she'd have someone else to share her frustration and shame with over her eldest daughter, and I could get away.

Of course, in actuality, his appearance wouldn't help. If my father happened to come in while she was chastising me, he'd take one look at the situation and hide in the kitchen.

Just another day in my world. At least my sister had diverted her attention this time. I maneuvered around my chirpy sibling and my entranced mother while they were busily discussing the glorious world of the petite and socially accepted.

Those days when Mother would use me for target practice, and her voice would finally get hoarse if no one came in to turn her attention elsewhere, I would patiently wait until she had exhausted herself. I would mumble something about how she was right. I was a disgrace and wouldn't get anyone to marry me and take me off her hands. She would be mollified, give me one more angry look and finally let me go.

When I'd get to my room, I'd drop the malicious plastic bags on my bed and join them for a moment, lying down so the girdle couldn't keep cutting me in the waist with its vicious silver claws. I'd reach through my clothes, grab it as it fought to deepen the raw red rivulets of skin running from the tops of my thighs to about halfway up my chest. I already had stretch marks as if I'd given birth a dozen times. The raised long lines of indentations after I removed the offensive girdle were permanent. They crawled up and down my abdomen like white worms implanted under my skin. Not a pretty sight.

Now that I was rested, I'd start wrestling the sadistic spandex off my butt to my legs and then onto the floor. If I had forgotten to cover the half mirror attached to the back of my door, I'd see combat between an overweight girl and what looked like an anaconda wrapped around her as she tugged, thrust her buttocks into the air, and grunted as she pulled the barbarous garment/anaconda off her. At least, I didn't have to see the torture marks on my legs, since the mirror stopped at a little past my middle.

I'd stop for a minute, transfixed by what I was seeing. Dirty blonde hair clinging like wet moss to a flushed round face, watery blue eyes squeezed almost shut, and about 160 pounds of inflated skin rumbling around beneath the surface of her shirt and skirt. No wonder Mother didn't love me. I was grotesque. Who could love a rolling fat wave of a person? Worse, it looked like I wasn't going to get any taller than my five feet, four inches so the layers of fat couldn't be spread over a taller frame. I didn't deserve to be loved. I had become the American nightmare for teenage girls. I was not pleasantly plumb with baby-fat chubby cheeks just waiting to be pinched by loving relatives; I wasn't just overweight and needed to lose a few pounds. Nope, I was fat on my way to obese. I was the "Before" picture in all the women's magazines. I couldn't ever pose for the "After" photo. I was doomed.

Then I'd start another emotional eating binge. I'd tell myself it didn't matter how I looked, anyway. Mother would always be ashamed of her behemoth daughter who waddled next to her when she would be forced to go outside of the house with me.

Such was life with my family when I was twelve

Well, that's a brief introduction to the beginning of my tale of how I became the social prey in a society that hunts down the most fragile of its members. I wanted you to meet my family and see where I was coming from, so you could understand where I have been. Now it's time to tell you my story. It's one that most girls and women can relate to. I don't "pull any punches" or "sugercoat" it. It's not easy to read, and it sure wasn't easy to write. But you need to see what I saw, feel what I felt, and learn what I didn't until the end. The beginning of my story I call "Fat Truths," the social rules that fat girls have to live with and sometimes die by.

I want you to be empowered by what I have to say, so you don't end up where I did. If you have a family member like me, it will let you see into her world. It's a real look at the most vulnerable among us, at how they are damaged and how they can be helped.

Chapter 2

"Fat Truths"

Fat girls will tell you the truth. They only lie to themselves. My fat-girl story doesn't have a happy ending. That's why I'm telling it to you now. My low self-esteem and "people-pleaser" behavior have led to a shortening of my life. Because I was starved for affection, I developed full-blown addictions to bulimia and amphetamines that lasted 15 years. They have had a devastating effect on my health. It is too late for me to get back those years. By sharing my story as a fat girl, I hope someone may benefit from my mistakes.

Fat girls have always been easy targets. They are society's pariahs. The people everyone gets a free shot at. From birth girls are judged on how they look. If you're taking up more room in your pink blanket than the boy in his blue one in the basinet next to you, you're in trouble. For a girl nothing matters more than her weight. When you're fat, you're dead in the water. Even worse than a beached whale that at least makes it to shore to die. Fat girls float belly up in society.

Nobody looks at them twice, unless they want to feel good about themselves or make fun of them.

"Jesus, did you get a look at her?"

"Yeah, if I was that fat I'd stay home."

Well, surely families of fat girls love them. Think again. Fat girls are walking billboards that proclaim to the world their mothers and fathers are bad parents. Siblings make their lives a living hell.

"C'mon, Mom, do I have to take bubble butt with me?"

"Hey, leave some food for the rest of us, Tank."

Fat girls have mothers who tell them to wear clean underpants in case they get in a car wreck.

"What if the ambulance men have to see underneath your clothes?"

Mothers of fat girls know what would happen.

"If they see dirty panties they'll believe you're a fat slob. Or worse, if they see the SIZE of your panties they'll think to themselves, 'How are we gonna get her on the stretcher? I didn't know girls could get so big.'" Such embarrassment.

When you're fat, even your own mother is ashamed of you. You can't even be hurt or die in peace out on the street. Some fat girl's mother is pointing and hollering, "See, I told you so!" when the fat girl's panties are exposed to the world.

Skinny people believe fat girls shouldn't have existed in the first place. Fat people have fat kids. Fat people shouldn't be allowed to breed. God, it's bad enough to have to see fat girls. Fat families are absolutely disgusting in every sense of the word. It should be a felony for them to appear in public. Fat girls are genetic mistakes. Fat cleansing of the population to destroy those with the fat gene should be instituted immediately. The economy will save on foodstuffs and the costs of clothing. Fat people eat all the food and drive up the prices of wearing apparel. Everything has to be made bigger to fit their gigantic bodies. Society suffers in so many ways by having fat people in it. If only they'd disappear.

I knew they were talking about me. I would make the weight go away so they would want me to live in their world. I would do anything for them to like me. And I did. I embarked on a journey to slow suicide through an eating disorder and drug abuse.

I'm here to tell you it wasn't worth it. My bones are thin because they are calcium-deprived. I don't go to the dentist for annual checkups anymore; he'll see the holes in my teeth from the stomach acid that has eaten away the enamel. My heart has an erratic rhythm from the years of amphetamines. I have a startle reflex like soldiers with post-traumatic stress because of the uppers I lived on instead of food.

My 15-year bulimic and amphetamine-addicted downward spiral was abetted by my perfectionism and obsessive-compulsive behavior. Like most smart, sensitive, fat girls I would have done anything to be accepted, even though I tried not to show it. I wanted to be loved. I could have easily died numerous times from a shredded esophagus or an amphetamine-induced heart attack. I didn't care. I'd meet my goal of becoming thin, or die in the attempt. Dying was the lesser of the two options.

Now, I know I have lost a year for every one I devoted to my secret weight-loss solutions. Some would say I was primed from birth to fall victim to a genetic disposition to self-destruct. You've met my mother.

Like Mother, Like Daughter

She was mentally ill. She used alcohol and prescription drugs for most of her adult life after suffering years of emotional abuse from her father. Instead of fairy tales, she would tell me pieces of her life story every day I was with her.

Her father, my grandfather, was an "old country" Germanic disciplinarian whose hatred for my mother began when his beloved wife died giving birth to her. My mother believed he never forgave her.

I remember her sitting on the edge of my bed each night, telling me stories about her childhood. Her stories were frightening. I thought she was trying to show me what happened to little girls who disobeyed their parents, by telling me what her father did to her if she displeased him. She never questioned his actions. I never questioned her reasons for reliving them with me.

The one that remains the most vivid had to do with the rats. Sometimes at the dinner table her father would suddenly get up from his tall chair at the head of the table, walk quickly to her chair, and grab her by the back of her neck. She would frantically try to think of what she had done wrong.

I can still recall the fear in her voice as she recounted what occurred.

"Barbara, did you do what I asked you to do?"

She knew she had disappointed him again in some way.

"Did you hear me? Look at me when I'm speaking to you."

His face would be blood red from anger. Mother discovered later her father was an alcoholic. Her stepmother had been having fights with him for years over his drinking. Of course, he denied he was drinking any more than any other man with his responsibilities would. He never drank at work. Home was another matter entirely. Although my mother didn't know it at the time, her father used to hit her stepmother if he "had a mean drunk on."

Mother said she had to be careful not to speak directly to him. He'd take it as a challenge. She replayed the conversation for me.

"Was it about candling the eggs after school? I had to stay late for choir practice. I told Mom. I got to the store as soon as I could, Father."

Her parents owned a small grocery store in their hometown of St. Petersburg, Florida. She had worked for her father since she was old enough to separate the good eggs from the bad.

Mother looked for help from her stepmother at the other end of the table.

"Harold, she did tell me she was going to be a little late. I thought I told you this morning."

"You were late because of that stupid choir? Singing is a waste of time. How will that help you get a job after high school?"

Her father didn't really expect an answer. He only asked rhetorical questions. He was the supreme ruler in the home. His word was law.

Mother said she knew she had made a mistake as soon as the words left her mouth.

"The choir director says I could get a scholarship to an arts college with my voice."

Her father didn't bother to answer. His fingers tightened around her neck. Mother said it was like being in a vise. He lifted her out of the chair.

"I think some time in the cellar will get rid of this nonsense and make you understand your duties to the store and your family."

Mother told me she would begin to scream and beg as he dragged her away from the table. Her father had told her there were rats in the cellar that would bite disobedient girls.

"Please don't put me in there! I'll be good!"

Mother described how she would cling to his leg as he pushed her through the cellar door and locked it. She would cower on the top stair and try not to look into the darkness below. Her father stored produce in the cellar so it was kept extremely cold. Sometimes when he would bring up a bag of potatoes, there would be a hole at the bottom of one side of the burlap where he said a rat had gnawed through it.

25

She would be kept in the cellar for hours. She said she squeezed her eyes shut, and listened for the sound of the rats coming up the stairs to get her.

By this time I was petrified, with my head buried under the covers. Mother would pat where my head should be, say goodnight and close my door. I was too afraid to get out of bed to open it a little to let in some of the light from the hallway. My father, who had wanted a boy for his firstborn, would chide me about being scared of the dark if he saw the door was open a crack.

When I got older, I asked Mother if she had wanted to go to the arts college to pursue a singing career. I knew she had a beautiful voice. My father told me he loved to hear her singing around the house before I was born. She had lots of solos in the church choir. Everyone would say how wonderfully she sang.

"I'm sure my father would have let me go, but I knew in my heart he didn't approve. So I went to a business school close to home instead."

Beaten down both emotionally and psychologically, Mother had a really low opinion of herself. When she would get compliments about her singing, she would avert her eyes from those of the admirer, and mutter something denigrating about herself. I would come to see those same deficiencies in myself.

Sick in the Head

Her mental illness became more apparent as she got older. All the things she had missed out on became a festering sore in her. She looked for a cause. She found it in me.

To escape her abusive home, she married at eighteen. She had me at nineteen, and I was the reason she had been deprived of the life she could have had, if she hadn't become pregnant so soon. In those days, postpartum depression hadn't been discovered. It just added to her already unstable mental state.

She "doctor-shopped" to get her tranquilizers and amphetamines. In the 50s and 60s, women who saw doctors for insomnia or anxiety were females with unknown, scary, emotional problems. Family physicians didn't want to hear their stories about constant crying, sleeplessness, frustration, and dissatisfaction with their lots in life. Most doctors were men. Women had emotional baggage that was untreatable. Mother got lots of prescriptions for drugs that sedated her, and ones that made her hyperactive. When her toleration for one drug negated its effectiveness, she'd make an appointment with a different doctor to get something new and more powerful. With her mental disease, drugs made a bad situation a whole lot worse for all of us. She had an endless supply of different drugs from several doctors who saw her for ten minutes, and then wrote scripts for drugs to get her out of their offices.

Initially, I think she was trying to get help. Then she got addicted. Not one doctor suggested she get psychological counseling. Men didn't need such things. Women were weak. Asking for therapy wouldn't have occurred to Mother. Her father would have scoffed at the very idea the mind could be sick. He didn't trust doctors and wouldn't see one, even when his liver began to fail from cirrhosis from the years of alcohol abuse.

There were no classes on sex or parenting in my mother's era. Mother bitterly told me she thought she had probably gotten pregnant on her wedding night. She went from her father's house to her husband's house. That was what young women did. If they didn't go to college to find their mate, they usually married the first man they had a relationship with. Girlfriends from school were relegated to their pasts. It was now time to grow up and be a wife and a mother. Her father had told her so. Her stepmother had said nothing.

She told me she didn't know how to be a mother. When she was stuck at home with me all day and I would cry, she'd get so frustrated she'd slap me. It seemed an odd thing to tell a ten-year-old, but she had talked to me more as her peer than her daughter since I was old enough to listen to her. It was probably an unhealthy way to grow up, but I didn't know anything different.

By the time I was twelve, the toll she took on me was showing in the weight I was gaining each month. I had no friends to ask over so I could engage in girl-talk. I soon discovered it was not a good idea to have anyone over, anyway. She had begun drinking heavily, and popping downers at night to sleep and uppers in the morning to get herself awake. I never knew what kind of mood she would be in when I got home from school. Instinctively, I must have known it was not a good place to bring people. I was the child of an alcoholic, though I didn't know that at the time. But I didn't hear other girls talking about finding airplane-sized bottles of vodka in their mothers' shoes. They didn't mention their mothers' angry outbursts at the most trivial things. The question, "How was your day?" could set her off. Maybe my home life wasn't the norm.

Some Serious Drinking

There are easygoing drunks and mean drunks. My mother was a mean drunk like her father. She'd yell at us for hours. The weekends were the worse. My father would get his .22 caliber rifle and 30-30 shotgun and go to the shooting range. Now that I think of it, it was probably not a good idea to have guns around the house. Anyway, I had nowhere to go. I became her primary target. When my father would return, she'd blame her bad mood on me. Before I could get upstairs, he'd catch me and punch me in the mouth so I had a "fat lip," because I had mouthed off to my mother and upset her.

If I made it to my room, I'd hear her castigating him for his inability to discipline me. I knew what was coming. I could hear him coming upstairs, with my mother screaming in his ear. He'd go into their bedroom, grab his leather belt, and with her right alongside, he'd walk in my room and tell me "to assume the position." I'd bend over, and he'd hit me on the back and butt with the belt until his arm got tired.

Stubbornly, I taught myself not to make a sound as he beat me. I would focus on the number of times he would hit me before his arm got tired. After the first few times when I sobbed and begged him not to hit me, I was quiet. The sound of the belt whizzing through the air and the slap of it on my skin were the only noises in the room. And that would really irritate my mother. I wasn't crying enough for what I had done to make her life miserable. Silent tears rolling down my cheeks obviously didn't count. She'd finally leave in a huff. My dad would follow her downstairs, after he put the belt back on the hook in his closet.

I'd think to myself, as I poured cold water on my thighs and buttocks before climbing painfully into bed, *they couldn't make me cry out loud*. It was my one small victory in the constant battle with Mother. I didn't blame my father, though. He was as much a victim as I was.

He wasn't a bad father. It was the age when the threat, "Wait till your father gets home," was the way people dealt with their kids if they misbehaved. My mother wouldn't leave him alone until he had punished me. I don't think he liked hurting me. It was the only way he could have peace in the house.

I wasn't old enough to understand how sick my mother was. Her rage could not be seen in public. No one could know she wasn't the perfect wife and mother. That was the traditional family lifestyle in those days.

Like her father, she never drank at work. She was the perfect employee. She never missed a day. She'd be the one who baked cakes and cookies for the people in her office. She'd plan the office parties. She'd give rides to anyone who needed to go anywhere.

Everyone loved my mother – her kindness, her generosity. She never forgot to get a gift for someone's birthday, or to bring snacks on Friday for the entire office. Often, she'd bake until the early hours of the morning. She'd have about four hours of sleep, but there would be tons of pies, cookies, and cakes to take in to the office. She never complained at work. She'd be the first one to volunteer to stay late. Mother would bring home cards saying how wonderful she was, how cheerful, how hardworking.

I thought she was happy at work. Surely she felt needed and respected. I thought she liked her co-workers and boss since she was always doing things for them. Not true.

I finally saw my mother as the quintessential hypocrite. Her self-esteem was non-existent. At home she would tell us how used and unappreciated she was. She was doing all the work while everyone else got more money and the credit. Her paranoia would get a boost from her drinking once she was behind closed doors. I was confused. Was I supposed to like or hate the people she worked with? What attitude could I take so she would love me?

My distrust and inability to let down my guard became the foundation of my own dysfunctional relationships. Being fat just exacerbated the problem and gave my parents something on which they could both agree. Family problems were one thing, but having an overweight daughter showed the world what lousy parents they were. It was a no-win situation for me. So I kept on eating. Food replaced love.

I could experience pleasure through eating rather than wait for someone to give me affection. I had lots of secrets I couldn't tell anyone. Food was my friend. Friendships are made from sharing and mutual affection. I didn't trust anyone. I had no one to care about outside my parents. And I could never be sure what they felt about me. I was sure no one cared about me. You couldn't believe anything anyone said, anyway. It would come back to hurt you if you let them in. They'd use it against you somehow. Since I was fat, people kept their distance. Couldn't I be loved for the inner me? Couldn't they see past the defenses?

Mother smiled at people and hated their guts. Her sickness created my skewed view of the world. Most therapists go into the profession because they are screwed up themselves. My future career was already decided.

The Two Mothers

Mother was two different people. To the outside world, she was the epitome of generosity and understanding. A goddess of kindness. Once she was inside her house, she had an entirely different persona.

Years later as an adult, I understood she was mentally ill. To an adolescent who needed her guidance and love, she was a conundrum, a frightening contradiction, a daily time bomb I frequently triggered.

After a day of cheerful obedience to what she saw as her expected role so she could get affection, she'd come home to her other world, where she could be her real self. She'd put down her purse and car keys on the kitchen table. Usually she'd have an empty cookie tin or cake plate from the goodies she had brought to work that morning. They would go flying into the sink. Then the litany of her woes would begin. My father would still be at work. I was the recipient of her raging lectures on the injustices she had suffered that particular day.

I'd eventually notice she was refilling her water glass from a container in the refrigerator a lot, as she stomped around the kitchen and living room. Of course, she had vodka in her glass. She liked it for her secretive drinks, because it didn't have any odor or color. For months I thought it was ice water, until my father and I started our ritual of pouring out any liquids she had hidden around the house, including those in plain sight in the fridge.

Finally she'd tire herself out, and the liquor would take effect. She'd collapse on the living room couch and fall asleep. I'd go to my room and do my homework, until my father came home and roused her to get dinner.

This scenario was repeated daily for several years. But things changed when her drinking accelerated. She had also begun going out with her girlfriend from work on Friday nights. She'd say it helped her relax to go out and enjoy herself one night a week. Her friend was at least ten years younger. Mother liked to think she was still youthful. She told me she'd never had her dating and party years, so she was going to do them now.

My father didn't object. It would be quiet for a couple of hours. He would hope she would keep her drinking under control, since she was out in public. What people thought of her meant everything to her. A domineering father had made her emotionally malnourished. She fed on others' approval, though she despised herself for needing it, and hated them for making her need it.

Mother would get enraged if we brought up the subject of her limiting her drinks, so we waited until she got home to see what shape she was in.

Several times it was the police who called. Their dialogue with my father was similar on those occasions. I could repeat it word for word. My father would sit on the couch with his head in his hands. I'd wait. Then he'd speak:

"They've got your mother down at the jail in the Drunk Tank. She got into an argument with one of the officers, so they arrested her. They said she's in no condition to come home tonight. I guess her friend left her there in the bar. When she came out to get in her car, the bartender was worried and came out after her. He wanted to call her a cab or call her home, but your mother got argumentative, so he went back inside and called the police. They arrived as she was trying to fit her door key into the car door to unlock the car. They offered to call someone at home to come and get her, but she got combative with them when they insisted she sit on the curb until they could get her a ride home."

Sometimes, he would talk out loud about what he could do.

"Maybe if she stays there overnight…"

When Mother drank, her nice persona disappeared. She became her father's daughter, when he drank heavily and got mean in the bars or at home with her stepmother.

The phone would ring again. We would exchange resigned glances as my father picked up the receiver. We both knew who it was. Everybody got one phone call. Usually she would sleep off enough of the alcohol so she was coherent enough to ask for her phone call.

I could hear her on the other end. She had to yell to be heard. The jails got pretty noisy at night when the drunks woke up.

"When are you coming to get me out of here?" She sounded angry, like it was our fault she was in a cell with puking junkies and raucous prostitutes.

"Well, I thought if you were there in the morning, you might get some help with this."

If my father tried this particular way of responding to her, she'd change her tone.

"I can't stay here. I don't belong in here with these people. I promise I'll get some help." She started crying.

I knew she had him then. My father would get up, put on his coat and look for his car keys. He'd turn to me as he was leaving.

"Now, it might take me a little while to get your mother home. Don't stay up. I'm sure she'll be fine in the morning."

I'd try to stay awake in case he needed me when he brought her home, but I'd usually fall asleep on the sofa. When the police didn't call late in the evening after the bars closed, we knew she was coming home on her own. I'd make sure to drink lots of soda full of caffeine so I could stay awake for what was inevitably going to happen.

It would be three in the morning sometimes when we would hear the gate creaking. When she slid the glass doors open, we could gauge what kind of situation we would be facing by the way she closed them. If she missed the latch completely and stumbled over the doorstep, it was going to be a rough time with her.

She'd usually have to go to the bathroom.

"Gotta pee."

She'd squat where she was. We'd have to move fast to get her to the bathroom in time. We'd each grab an arm and pull her up. She was so drunk she was dead weight at this point. If she slumped into a squat again, she'd urinate on the carpet. My father would give me an embarrassed look and ease her down to the floor.

"Looks like she can't hold it. I'll clean it up later."

Those times we got her to the downstairs bathroom, I'd have to quickly get her clothes off so she didn't pee all over them. I'd hold her upright on the toilet, while my father stood outside the open door.

"C'mon, Mom, let's get you upstairs to bed."

I wiped her dry, pulled up her pants, and we maneuvered her up the stairs into their bedroom. Dad would pull her up on the bed and cover her. She'd start snoring. He'd go back downstairs, and I'd go to bed. During most of my adolescence, this was our Friday night ritual in the 1960s.

My father and I didn't talk about these sessions. I think it was too painful for him to discuss. I just assumed this was how other families lived. I guess I wasn't dealing with it, because instead of alcohol to cover my emotional pain I used food.

Before Mother would load up her car with her office baked goods, I'd sneak handfuls of cookies or often a complete pie or cake to take to my room. I'd gorge and then get ready for school. My school clothes were getting pretty snug, but I had some old sweaters that came down to my knees. The fat would be hidden, for the time being. Actually, I was acting out another genetic trait.

Physical Deformity

The female bodies in our home had one strike against them from the time we reached puberty. Something else that ate at my mother was her legs. She had a beautiful face and a lovely singing voice, but her legs embarrassed her. My mother had fat legs, but was normal on top. I don't mean her legs were a little heavy. They looked like they were in the early stages of elephantitis. We would have fit in quite nicely posing for the painter Peter Paul Reuben in the leg department, except we weren't voluptuous; we just had the huge legs. I inherited her body structure. I was thin until I hit puberty. I have a picture of me standing on some rock, thin arms hanging at my sides, thin legs strong-looking on top of the rock. I am smiling. That is the last time I was a regular-sized girl. And I stopped smiling.

The girdles came first. If you have ever seen those old catalogs showing those monstrous corsets for women, you can get some idea of what it was like suffering in a girdle at twelve. No one talked about dieting back in my mother's day. We both thought we would just have to live with our fat legs. But she knew about girdles since she had been locked into them by her father, who was embarrassed to take her out in public the way she was.

I remember her hauling me to the lingerie department for my first training bra. It didn't take her long to choose a formless white bra for me. Then the important garment came next. This would take some time. The girdles were in the women's section, far away from the "girl's-first-training bra" tables in the front. The girdles were heavy so you couldn't hang them on those small hangers like they used for delicate lingerie. I later thought that anything under ten pounds was "delicate lingerie."

The first question to the saleslady pinpointed the time in my life when things started to go dark:

"Do you have girdles for heavy teens?"

The saleslady looked me up and down. I stood there like one of those Budweiser horses ready for harnessing. Actually, after the girdle pages in the old catalogs, the horses' harnesses were on the next several pages.

"Yes, we have some on the back table there." She pointed in some vague direction to some recess in the back of the large-panties section.

My mother pulled me towards the table laden with large, cruel-looking white things with ugly clasps attached to the leg portions. I guess the manufacturers thought, "Once a fat girl, always a fat woman," so they planned ahead for when she would need to wear hose.

Mother sorted through them for a bit, selected several that looked indistinguishable from the others, thrust them into my arms, and led me to the dressing rooms.

Oh no, she was coming in the dressing room with me.

I hadn't dressed or undressed in my mother's presence since I turned twelve. Maybe the horror of her helping me put on my first menstruation pad in the bathroom had done her in. What should have taken a couple of minutes took quite a while. Because of the burgeoning fat on my stomach, butt, and thighs, it was next to impossible to attach the pad to the metal clasps. The whole apparatus kept getting lost in the fat folds. She had to lift up the fat shelf of my stomach first.

"Now put your hands here, so I can see the hooks on the belt." The elastic started to come alive and snap everywhere when she tried to attach anything to it.

"Pull your legs apart so I can see the pad. I think I see it!" It felt like she had found the lost kingdom in those Indiana Jones movies. She grappled with the hook and the pad for what seemed like forever, as I stood there like a slaughtered cow. I had to keep holding my stomach out of the way, while keeping a bath towel in place to wipe up the blood dripping down the insides of my thighs. I felt like I was in my own horror film. It was nothing like I imagined "becoming a woman" would be like. This was messy, frustrating and grotesque. Finally, I heard a sigh of relief from my nether area as my mother stood up and regarded what she had accomplished.

"That should do it. You'll have to change it when it gets soaked." With that last bit of motherly advice, she was out the door before I could ask her anything about this contraption. It was making an angry-looking, red indentation around my abdomen. Its nasty hooks were stabbing me in the front and back of my thighs.

I sat down on the lid of the toilet to see between my legs. The metal clasps were putting up a losing fight to hold onto the cloth ends of the sanitary napkin. It had turned sideways and was caught between my butt cheeks. I spread my legs as far as I could, without doing permanent damage to them by hitting the sink and bathtub on either side of the toilet. My knees took a beating, though, as I stretched and squirmed to get the pad sorted out. I had this fear of it tearing loose from the metal clamps, and getting lost between my thighs. Of course by the time I'd gotten everything battened down, the pad needed changing.

Anyway, that was the last time my mother saw me undressed. She'd knock on the door or holler up the stairs, but she didn't come into my room until I left for college. She said it was to give me privacy and independence. I think she was worried she'd have to help me with something else distasteful that would remind her what a chore it was to have an overweight daughter.

Since I didn't have any girlfriends to ask about this menstruating thing, I didn't know until I was a freshman in college and saw some boxes of tampons in the communal bathrooms, that there was a less cumbersome way to handle this female problem each month. Another heavyweight on my floor explained what to do with the paper tube. It took a box to get it right, but what a relief not to have to use that awful elastic belt with those horrific metal monsters digging into my flesh.

But that was nothing compared to the actual gut-wrenching agony of cramps I'd get at "that time of the month." I thought I would die. I *wanted* to die! They were so bad I'd curl up in a fetal position on my bathroom floor and moan. I lived on aspirin so I could go to school. I would gobble handfuls of any over-the-counter painkillers I could get my hands on. So this awful painful event each month was so I could have kids? Whose idea was that? Oh yeah. Eve punished for her sin. The rest of us along with her.

I dreaded my periods like the plague. Probably being bitten by rapid bats would have been less painful. Since I was fat, I thought it highly unlikely I'd get anyone to have kids with me anyway. *God must have it in for girls*, I thought, *especially fat girls.*

When I first saw the ugly big silver snaps on the girdle, I knew God was thinking out loud, "Round Two, Tubby, let's see what ya got."

We didn't have full-length mirrors in our home, just the half ones that made the rooms look bigger. Even the one on the back of my door didn't show all of you. It stopped at mid-thigh. This was the first time I would see myself from top to bottom. As I struggled into the first girdle, my attitude changed for the worse. I looked ridiculous and felt awful.

"Mom, why do I have to wear this? It doesn't feel comfortable at all."

Mother surveyed me like a territory yet to be named. She looked at me in the girdle in the mirror, and pulled it higher up on my waist.

"It's not supposed to feel good, but it works. You want to have nice clothes for school, don't you? Well, this is how we're going to get you into some decent outfits."

Satisfied that she had found the right one, we both struggled to pull it off me. Looking in the mirror as this fight to release me from my first Iron Maiden was taking place, I felt ashamed of what I was seeing. Why was this happening? Why couldn't I find clothes that didn't need this instrument of torture? What was wrong with the way I looked?

Chapter 3

Not What I Want to Hear

Mother answered all my questions:

"You'll just have to get used to being big down there. There's nothing we can do about it."

That was the last time for years that I looked into a full-length mirror anyplace, or even glanced in a store-front window that reflected my appearance back to me. I was different from the rest of the pubescent population of females. It was the worst thing that could happen to girls who idolized Barbie dolls. I was heavy, overweight, big "down there." It didn't matter that my top was normal; I was big where it counted most for social acceptance. My butt and thighs would be my curse. I would be socially shunned. For a girl about to become a teenager and take on the world, I got my first and last lesson about what people wanted to see. It wasn't fat girls. The world didn't want me. Girls would snicker; boys wouldn't ask me out. I was crushed.

When I got home, I took the offensive garment up to my room, threw it in a mostly empty panty drawer, got out my stash of milk chocolate bars, and ate at least five. I slid the wrappers under my mattress.

I found that it didn't do any good to feel sorry for myself. As soon as I started protesting about my lot in life, my mother would scold me:

"That's just the way we're built. We just have to make the best of it. Now clean your plate."

Mother always told me to clean my place. There were those starving children in some Third World country who would give anything to have food like this.

Well, I thought bitterly, *they're better off than I am. If they're starving, the girls have skinny legs and no butt.* Irrational and highly insensitive, I know. But that's how I felt, as I scooped up the last mound of mashed potatoes and stuffed them into my mouth.

Fat Girl at Play

My social life started rather inauspiciously. But then again, what can you expect for a fat girl. It began like many little girls - with scouting. And scouting started out well for me. When I was young, I was a Brownie. I was cute and slender in my little dun-colored uniform. There is an old photo of me looking just like every other six-year-old, with my precious Brownie beret perched jauntily on my head. But you can't be a Brownie forever. When you hit puberty, you have to move up.

Most little girls like puberty. You lose the baby fat and start thinking about boys. You gossip about them and other girls for hours on end. Those tank tops and tiny shorts are just waiting to be worn.

You remember what happened when I hit puberty. Well, no surprises here then.

Yeah, I turned into the Incredible Hulking Girl Scout. There are no pictures of me as a Girl Scout. I knew why.

The uniforms were two-parters. The two parts came together in one package. You couldn't buy them separately. So there I was, normal on top and gargantuan on the bottom. Girdles and pantyhose were my basics rather than merit badges. I looked awful, anyway. The olive-green skirt was so tight I could barely walk. I carried safety pins in my pockets in case the thread came loose, and I leaked out like bread dough. If I tried to sit, the skirt made an unnatural journey up my legs. The girdle straps would become visible, as they bit into my upper thighs and the backs of my legs. My socks with the **GS** logo were the nylon kind that gripped my calves like tourniquets. Usually I would surreptitiously push them down, so my circulation wasn't cut off completely. The belt had a neat gold-medal **GS** on it where it came together. Since my stomach fat kind of obliterated my waist when I sat down, the **GS** buckle was crushed into my flesh like a hot-iron tattoo.

Unfortunately, the badge sash wasn't big enough or long enough to cover anything below my waist. As a perfectionist, I earned every badge. As a fat girl, I hoped there were some big badges that might stretch over the sash, to cover some of the fat below my waist. No such luck. And those badges were SO colorful. Great. People would be attracted to the neon colors and look at the wearer. Expressions of curiosity and admiration quickly became ones of distaste and disdain. The comments were equally as hurtful.

"Don't they have a weight limit for Girl Scouts?"

"Jesus, did she miss the badge on nutrition?"

"Now I know what the Jolly Green Giant would look like as a Girl Scout."

But the annual Girl Scout Camp each summer was free, so my parents had some place to send me out of the neighborhood. I think they hoped the required hikes would bring them back a svelte teenager, rather than Beulah the Beluga Whale. So the summer before I went to high school, I had my first grown-up social experience.

I remember the camp was located in some heavily wooded areas with enormous trees. Along with the foliage, there were innumerable insects that bit every available square inch of your body. They had a veritable feast every day and night on mine. I'd build roaring fires that would incinerate any marshmallows or scouts who got too close, but I thought they'd keep off the bugs. I'd usually be sitting around them by myself, anyway, singing *Kumbaya,* while the others congregated in various tents, where they gossiped about boys, clothes and other girls. I was never invited to join them. They probably thought I had no friends to talk about. No boys would be interested in me. They had seen me in my Girl Scout uniform, so I definitely knew nothing about clothes. So I was ostracized. Welcome to the new social world of the fat girl. I should have stayed home. I was used to being criticized and ignored there. I didn't have to let the rest of the world start in on me, too.

Well, I wasn't a "group person," anyway. Unfortunately, everything at camp was designed for groups.

There was even a communal shower. All these slim girls would go in, take off their towels, and gracefully revolve in the water like baby seals. At least I thought that's what they did. I didn't care whether they floated ethereally through the spray like Disney mermaids. I didn't want to see them, or be in the same place where comparisons could be made on any level of physical appearance. The only way to avoid the communal shower was to have your period, so you could use the adult camp counselor's shower. It had canvas tent walls that closed you off from view. I was the only girl who had a period for the entire summer. But maybe the counselors didn't want to look at me, either, because they never called me on the never-ending menstruation. They must have thought my suitcase was filled with more Maxi-pads than clothes.

I thought the one physical activity where I might be on a par with the rest of the natural athletes in that camp was in swimming. You know what they say about fat girls and water. They float extremely well.

You had to pass the swimming test in order to be allowed out past the knee-deep water that was close to the shoreline. I knew I could excel here. When I got so fat I couldn't get anyone to take me to the community pool, I'd take the bus there in the evenings when all the old people came in for their water aerobics. They'd be at one end of the pool leaping up and down like so many senile hippos, and I'd be swimming at the other. It was so peaceful. When I'd swim underneath the surface, I couldn't hear anything but the bubbles escaping from my lungs. I was graceful in the water. I propelled myself gently down the lane, kicking my feet and doing half-arm snow angel movements. Those were some of the happiest moments of my life.

And now at camp I'd get to be one of the girls, for once. I could swim with the best of them. I would excel at the swimming test. All my campmates would be envious, and say nice things where I could hear them. Mother would have been so proud.

On the morning of the test, I was dressed in my enormous, one-piece Ali Baba swimsuit, and had wrapped my bottom half in a huge beach towel. I had packed an over-sized swim cap and goggles. I had purchased some men's swim throngs. I was ready.

The camp's loudspeaker came on.

"Everyone report to the lake for the swimming test."

I held back so "the thins" could get ahead. If I were in front of them, I'd be sure to hear their derogatory comments.

"Hey, look up ahead. Did she think this was a fat camp?"

"My two sisters *together* don't have that big an ass."

"I hope she leaves some water for the rest of us when she jumps in."

What did that anorectic bimbo mean – when 'she jumps in?' I thought we'd swim out to the lifeguards, past the buoys I had seen on the lake when we arrived at the campsite. I remembered the buoys had Girl Scout logos painted on their sides.

I was thinking, *they'd be easy to see. It shouldn't take me long to get there, see the lifeguards give a 'thumbs up' signal to me, and turn around to swim back. I'd masterfully swim past those skinny, bikini-clad, blow-up dolls struggling to keep their heads out of the water, so they didn't mess up their expensive makeup. Stupid thins. I'd have the last laugh this time. When I get to the man-made beach first, I bet they give me a swimming merit badge on the spot.*

I chuckled to myself. The airheads looked back at the sound, found it was me making it, and kept their conversations going, as if they hadn't seen a thing – certainly nothing to disrupt their loud gossip.

I arrived at the lake and saw something happening at the end of the pier that extended out into the lake. Two lifeguards were standing on either side of the end of the pier. They were looking down into the opaque water.

Aren't we all gonna line up on the shore and then swim out? What are they doing at the end of the pier? I'm definitely not feeling good about this, I worriedly thought to myself.

The thins are walking down to the end. I'm behind them. As I get closer to the lifeguards, I see the thins get in a line I hadn't noticed. They're complaining about something, but I can't hear them until I get at the end of the line.

"This is ridiculous. Why can't they just take our word for it we can swim, for God's sake."

"Yeah. Most of us have home pools where we had private lessons. I remember this one guy my parents hired one summer. He was so hot."

"Well, if I have to jump in and float for a few minutes, at least I'll get to flirt with those babe lifeguards first."

This did not bode well for me. I didn't want *to jump in* anything. I wanted to swim out to the buoys, make a great turn, and then swim back with a triumphant smile on my chubby cheeks. I would look good in the water. It disguised my weight. If I had to jump from a height, I'd look like the Titanic sinking. Only there wouldn't be any Leo or band playing. I'd be an enormous torpedo with wings. My suit would catch the draft. The ruffled skirts sewed on the chest and waist would be like an obscene parachute attached to me. Not an attractive sight.

Maybe I could talk them into letting me swim out from the shore. I could tell them I'm afraid of heights.

Crap. This line is really moving.

It was my turn. I had hung back, so I was the last to go. Everyone else had jumped in, and swum back to the beach. As there was nothing to see on the beach because the lifeguards were still on the pier, all eyes focused on me.

Just peachy.

I stepped out of my throngs and laid my towel on top. At least, I didn't have far to walk. The line had gone all the way to the end.

The Keanu Reeves-looking lifeguard on my left gestured for me to come forward. I looked down. It was about a 20-foot drop, for crissakes. Who the hell thought this up? Definitely not a fat girl.

"Just put your feet on the edge, take a breath, and let go."

Right. Easy for him to say.

I couldn't even see my feet, as I scrunched my toes to hold onto the end of the pier.

"When you land, we'll see how you handle the deep water. If you can tread water, you'll be fine," said the Leonardo di Caprio-looking lifeguard on my right.

The thoughts rushed through my head.

*Don't they have any ugly lifeguards? These guys look like they acted on **Baywatch**. And I'm no Pamela Anderson, by a long stretch. Maybe I could tell them...*

While I was trying to think of an excuse why I couldn't jump off the pier, the two lifeguards put a hand on each side of my back and pushed. I lost my balance and landed on my stomach in the water. It hurt like hell. The splash was so high the lifeguards got soaked. I flailed in the water like a whale on steroids. And then it got worse. I started to sink. I got a mouthful of water, so I was gasping for air as I was going down.

Oh no! Just let me drown.

Both lifeguards had jumped in, and were trying to grab some part of me before I hit the bottom of the lake. *Humiliating* didn't even come close to describing what was happening.

I pulled away from them as hard as I could, but they had a death grip on me. I finally gave up, and they did a two-person rescue swim with me back to the beach.

By that time, my face was bright red. My suit had ridden up on my butt, so the fat looked like chum to draw sharks. I couldn't see a thing. My goggles had come off when I slammed into the water.

As I was hauled onto the beach like a huge, overturned sailboat, I heard the giggles from the thins.

Terrific.

Two of the female camp counselors leaned over me and said, "You'll have to stay in the shallows when everyone is swimming."

It turned out it was just me and some other fat chick that didn't know how to swim at all, that were restricted to the shallows.

Well, maybe no one would notice. Oh wait. They used a permanent marker to put a gigantic red X on my suit, so the lifeguards could make sure I stayed out of the deep water.

That day just couldn't get any worse. Oh yeah, it could.

The camp loudspeaker blared:

"Tomorrow we go on our first hike. Make sure you bring lots of water for the climb!"

Finally camp ended, and I climbed on the bus to go home. It was the only climbing I did at camp. I had lots of stomachaches at precisely the times of the hikes. The counselors didn't push it. Maybe they were worried they'd have to baby sit me the whole way.

I had a seat to myself. Nobody talked to me. I absentmindedly scratched the welts on my legs for the next two hours.

At least the bugs knew I'm alive, I thought sadly.

All the parents were waiting in the parking lot of the local church for the bus to arrive. I waited until everyone else had gotten off, been greeted and hugged, and was on their way out of the lot.

When I finally stepped off the bus, Mother took one long look at me. She didn't say a word, but heaved an enormous sigh as she walked ahead of me towards the car. I followed mutely behind, lugging the dirty green Girl Scout tote with all the badges inside I had earned – more than anyone else. The other girls were more interested in socializing than working for badges. I had nothing else to do.

When we got home, I trudged up to my room and threw the canvas bag on the floor.

I regarded myself in the mirror in my room. My skin was red and blotchy; I knew my arms and legs were swollen from bug bites, and my hair was plastered to my face. *Gross*.

I was glad I had waited until all the other girls had left the bus.

Mother hollered from downstairs.

"Bring your dirty clothes to the laundry room after you take a shower."

My bright-green canvas Girl Scout bag smelled like a busload of wet socks. An apt description. Seems the humidity had caused mold to grow on my underwear, shirts, and shorts.

I spent 45 minutes in the shower, letting the hot water run over me and feeling sorry for myself. The pain in my arms and legs from the open bug-bite sores was nothing compared to what I felt inside.

I threw my moldy Girl Scout uniform in the trash with my swimsuit.

It took three weeks for my arms and legs to heal. I had white calamine lotion smeared all over them. I resembled one of those tribes that paints itself white to scare its enemies.

"Jesus, she looks like a giant infected moth." My father was nothing if not candid about how he felt.

That night, with my fat, calamine-smeared legs stuck out in front of me, I closed my eyes.

As I nodded off, I thought, *maybe high school will be a place I can fit in.*

Eat and Be Eaten

It's a good thing I have a razor-sharp wit and am pretty smart, or I wouldn't have had even acquaintances in high school, much less friends. Being in the honor classes with other odd-looking girls and boys made my life bearable among the majority of kids in high school who enjoyed tormenting me. Even skinny ugly girls could make fun of me. Teachers in regular classes who needed an easy target would find one if I was in their classes. I would be scrunching around in my dress that was riding up my thighs, trying to keep my girdle from chafing the tender skin between my legs. The usual idiots would snicker, as they watched me try to keep my inner thighs from looking like raw meat.

"What's the problem?"

The in-bred dumbasses would shut up just as she turned from the blackboard. The only movement she would catch from her peripheral vision would be me, attempting to remain as still as possible now. Seldom worked.

"Can't you sit still?"

She would glare unmercifully at me for a moment, then turn back to what she was writing on the chalkboard. So much for adult empathy.

The classroom furniture was against me, too. Some skeletal freak decided that school desks should fit those perfect blonde-girl butts. The boys were supposed to lounge all over, so it didn't matter how they sat or sprawled at their desks. But for me, desks were another sign that the world wasn't built for doublewide. I bet those desk guys also make airplane seats in Coach.

"Take your seats, everyone." The boys moved fast to get the ones in the back. I usually ended up in the second row behind the ever-present cheerleader, who always sat in front in her name-brand clothes that fitted her perfectly. It didn't help that on Fridays, "School Colors Day," she wore her cheerleading outfit, with the short skirt just barely covering those perfectly formed legs. Even the short cheerleaders had proportionate legs. Nobody would cheer for a fat cheerleader, so I never saw one on the squad.

It didn't help that the school colors were yellow and white. Fat girls looked like large cobs of corn on Fridays, no matter what clothing combination they tried to wear to be part of the crowd. A fat girl was a crowd by herself. You can be dumb as a brick, poor as a homeless person, thin as a comb, but you can't be fat. It's the worst sin there is in high school. Even kids with acne that made you puke when you looked at them, were accepted over fat girls. You could look at their clothes instead of their faces when you talked to the acne freaks, but with fat girls there wasn't any place that wasn't fat.

I remember my first school assembly. In fact, I looked forward to it. I wouldn't have gym class that afternoon, one of the banes of my existence. Even though I looked like an overripe corncob, I had carefully chosen school colors to show my love for my school. Well, maybe not love. It was more like "I-have-to-be-here-so-I'll-try-to-make-the-best-of-it" sentiment.

Anyway, when the loudspeaker blared, "Everyone go to the gymnasium for the fall assembly," I made my way almost happily to my first high school assembly. As I entered, I saw that the gym had different sections for each class. Gazing at the mostly little skinny bodies of the boys and girls sitting under the Freshmen banner, I muttered to myself, "Jeez, they all look like elementary school kids. I'm gonna stand out like a sore thumb." One of Mother's favorite phrases to use against me. I now regretted that I probably looked like a neon unshucked cob of corn in my white blouse and yellow skirt - school colors be damned!

Well, maybe if I sit on the bottom row, I won't be so noticeable.

I found a place at the end of the freshmen section row on the bottom near the aisle between the sophomores and us. Bad move.

My yellow-covered skirt thigh extended into the aisle. I grabbed handfuls of my skirt and pulled them towards my lab. Now, I probably looked like some country western dancer clogger with bouffant crinoline layers of skirt thrusting out towards the gym floor.

Crap, crap, and double crap.

The freshman football team was heading towards my aisle to sit under the banner. As they ran up the metal steps, it sounded like a herd of buffalo terrorized by Indians on horseback. All eyes from both sections went to where the noise was coming from. Naturally, the fat girl desperately holding the sides of her skirt together in her lap was the first thing they saw. Teenagers aren't usually reticent about their feelings or thoughts.

"Oh my God! Who's that girl sitting near the floor? What's she doing with her skirt?"

Sophomores, who think they know everything since they survived their freshman year, are particularly known to be smart-asses with the sensitivity of elephant hide.

"She's not a freshman, is she? I've never seen one that big!"

"Go down and ask her."

Oh please don't let him come down – please, please, please. God, I'll do anything.

If God was keeping a tab on the times I had promised him I'd do anything, he must have run out of celestial paper by now.

Fortunately, the assembly was starting and we all had to stand for the Pledge of Allegiance. I thought I'd be safe now.

Of course not, what was I thinking?

Spit wads were landing on the back of my neck and in my hair. I didn't dare turn around to see who was doing it. They'd love that. So when I sat down, I clutched my skirt in one fist and tried unobtrusively to pick the gobs of paper saliva off my neck and out of my hair with the other

When the dance team danced their skin-tight leotard selves onto the floor, the cretins stopped abusing me and started nudging each other about the size of each girl's breasts while dancers undulated down the length of the gym. It looked more like pole dancing moves than actual dancing. So much for subtle choreography.

I relaxed as I heard the principal take the microphone to welcome all of us to our first high school fall assembly. He then turned the proceedings over to the head of the student council who began calling up the captains of the athletic teams to introduce their sport and their teams.

I could even feel myself smiling as I looked at the seniors on the teams. Those were some big, good-looking jocks! I knew the prom queens, dirty dance crew, and the ever-irritatingly, perfect cheerleaders had them, but I could dream, couldn't I?

With the band belching loudly and off-key from one side of the gym and the cheerleaders leading a "cheer-off" in front of each section, I was actually enjoying the whole high school assembly thing. And then they started the games in the middle of the floor. The captains of the athletic teams were supposed to pick people from the stands to participate.

Never happen. I can't be *that* unlucky!

Oh, crap.

The captain of the school soccer team was heading in my direction to choose someone to do the game with him. He'd never make it past the cheerleaders screaming in front of my bleachers. I wasn't even paying attention to what the game *was*, since I absolutely knew I wouldn't be chosen. I never got picked for anything. Even in elementary school, I was usually the last to be foisted off on someone for team sports during recess.

Damn. He's coming closer. Can I get up to leave? I'll tell the teacher guards at the gym doors I'm not feeling well. Something about the noise giving me a migraine. Okay, here goes!

Hold on a sec. I'm in luck.

He was stopped by one of the golden goddesses who managed to wrap herself sinuously around him.

"Brandon, how about we meet after the game Friday night? I've got something to show you." She looked like she was actually eating his ear with her lips pressed against it. And I could imagine what she had to show him. Sad to say, I'd have to imagine any kind of pubescent sex since the reality of it would not pause at my stop in life.

I concentrated on the girl at the microphone in the front of the gym. I wasn't too excited about hearing Brandon's response.

I looked around to see if anyone was heading down the bleachers aisle to join the hunk on the floor.

Someone was leaning over me. Evidently, Brandon had spent so much time with the dimwit cheerleader, he had to get someone fast.

"I pick you. C'mon."

You've got to be kidding me.

I felt a tug on my arm. Suddenly, I was almost airborne as the muscled jock pulled me into the center of the gym floor to join the other pairs of athletes and bleacher participants.

This can't be happening. I'm living a nightmare.

They were explaining the rules, but I didn't hear a thing.

"Look, maybe you could get someone else," I yelled in the soccer star's ear.

Ohmygod, they're putting an egg under his chin.

"Now each pair will exchange the egg all the way down the floor to our judges at the far end. Are you ready?"

No, no, no, I'm not....

The Adonis jock was turning his head for the exchange.

As he put his head next to mine, I thought, *Just my luck. I get someone like him this close, and he's trying to put an egg under my chin.*

His breath on my cheek would have been in my dreams for the whole year, but *this* was definitely not what I want to remember.

The egg dropped into one of my fat folds, and I felt myself moving down the floor. We were in first place since I could probably hold the egg like that until the damn thing hatched.

I attempted to lift my chins so he could get it from me. He was having a tough time finding it.

Just great. The entire school is watching while I make a fool of myself.

Other couples were going past us. We were stopped until he could get the egg from me to him.

Please, please, please, I'll do anything...

I hoped my old standby of desperate pleading would save me.

Yes, yes, yes!

I could feel the egg freeing itself and rolling towards his chin. This would be my shining moment. Everyone would know I had helped one of the school's best athletes win this contest. I would be popular. All the girls would want to know how it felt to be that close to one of the school's most handsome boys.

"Were his eyes really that blue?" "Did he smell good?"

I better pay attention, I thought, *so I can have my answers ready.*

Then it happened. The egg was stuck. It had rolled from one of my fat chins to the other and not to his. It was like superglue held it in place. Brandon looked like a hyperextended- necked turkey as he rammed his chin into what he took for my throat.

I could tell he was getting a might testy:

"Where the hell is it? Did you swallow the damn thing?"

Fearful of getting totally incapacitated by his chin butt, I moved my head desperately to the other side. Then I felt it. It was going to hit the gym floor.

"For chrissakes, you made us lose!"

We were the only two people standing in the middle of the gym, with the crushed egg between us on the floor. For a moment, there was absolute silence. Even the bad band and the pesky perky cheerleaders were quiet.

Ah, a touch of sympathy – a respite from verbal cruelty, a timeout from habitual abuse.

What were you thinking! Of course not.

The next five minutes were some of the longest of my miserable life. The laughter went on and on until it peaked in a shriek from the girl at the microphone. She was actually screaming into the mic.

"OH MY GOD! Can you believe that? That has to be the funniest…"

The soccer star gave me one last look of disgust and stomped away to threaten his team with a severe personal beating if they didn't stop laughing.

I stumbled back and hit an eggshell. My feet left the floor and all I could see was my voluminous, school-colored, ghastly yellow skirt in my face. Now some of the students were crying and holding their stomachs from laughing so hard.

Nobody came to help. The teachers were sitting among the students and vainly attempting to quiet them.

I got to my knees, then one knee with a hand supporting me on the floor and pushed myself up to a standing position. With as much dignity and self-composure I could muster, I patted down my skirt and made for the nearest exit. As I left, I could still hear the teachers shouting for quiet, but the entire student body was in an uproar.

I made my way to the school office and called Mother to come get me. It was like adding insult to injury when she would interrogate me on the way home, but at this point, I just needed to get away from the afternoon classes. I knew what would happen.

"Hey, are you that girl at the assembly?"

I couldn't put my head down on my desk since my upper body fat got in the way.

They would snicker and exchange unflattering remarks.

What other kind did I get?

"That's her. She fell on her ass. Jesus, it was SO funny."

"She looked like some fat duck stuck upside down."

Nope, even Mother was better than the savage verbal attacks I'd get in my classes. And my classes were anything but tolerable, anyway.

Every day was a battle with the small desks, the uncaring teachers, and the hateful kids.

Now, I don't want you to think I gave up and didn't make any social efforts to enjoy myself during my high school years. They not only had assemblies, they had school dances. And one was for freshmen only. I thought I'd give it a try. I was sure they kept the lights down low, and the music would be so loud people couldn't talk, especially about me.

They announced the Freshmen School Fling at the end of September. The school assembly debacle had died down. Most kids ignored me now. Maybe I'd make some friends at a social affair. I knew Mother would like that. She had stopped asking me each day if I had made any new friends at school.

The freshmen dance was on a Friday. I told Mother on Monday of that last week in September.

She was mixing batter in the kitchen.

"Mother, I think I'll…"

"Hey, hand me that bag of chocolate pieces."

Crap.

She was going to heft the bag and know many of the chocolate drops were missing. She'd see the little hole at the bottom of one side and the accusations would start.

I grabbed the bag, threw its diminished contents into the mixing bowl, and took her spoon from her to mix in the chocolate.

"Watch what you're doing. This cake has to be perfect. It's Boss Appreciation Day tomorrow. Everyone will stand around and sing, 'For he's a jolly good fellow' while they look at my cake."

"Sorry, Mom, I just thought I'd give you a hand. By the way, I thought I'd go to the Freshmen School Fling on Friday."

She actually stopped whipping the chocolate-flecked batter for a minute to look up at me.

"Did someone ask you to go? Is he in one of your classes? What's his name?"

"No, Mother, this is a dance where you can go by yourself and meet new freshmen who probably don't know everybody yet."

"Hmm. Not as good as a date, but at least you're going."

She bent her head over the deep bowl again.

"We'll have to get you something to wear. All you have is that dress you wore to your 8th grade promotion ceremony." She scrutinized my ballooning figure.

"Well, we know that won't fit anymore. I'll put this in the oven and we'll sit down and plan everything out."

This sounded like D-Day for World War II.

"I can just make a list of things I …"

"No, no, this might be your only chance to meet someone. Everything has to be just right. Go get some paper and a pen." She dusted the flour from her hands, popped the cake in the oven, set the timer, and turned back to me.

We sat down at the kitchen table to organize my social plan of attack.

"Now does this dance have a theme?"

"I don't think so. It's just for new freshmen."

"Okay then. Do you think there will be lots of lights?"

I could guess what she was thinking. Should we go dark with the dress or light? It depended on whether I was in full lights or could find some shadowed alcoves to move back in. Especially if there were lots of boys. Getting a good look at me in the harsh lights could be disastrous for snaring one.

"It's in the school gym, but I think they lower the lights once the dance begins."

"Damn, those rotten gym lights are so bright. Well, when I drop you off, stay outside until you hear the music for the first dance."

"We'll get your hair and nails done, too."

"Mom, I don't want to make a big deal out of this."

"It is a big deal. This is your chance to meet some nice young man. You could go on your first date!"

Each day was another step in the battle plan. By Friday night, I had everything in place for my entrance for the dance.

When I looked into the half-mirror on my closet door, I said out loud, "Not bad. Not bad at all."

Mother came in and stood at the door.

"Turn around. I want to make sure it doesn't bunch at the back. And for God's sake, stand up straight. You don't want to look like a hump-backed camel."

The dress passed muster. It was a bright blue that matched my eyes. It was cinched at the waist with a darker blue belt. Mother had added a few extra holes in it. It still felt a little tight, but it was definitely better than when I first put it on at the Big Women shop in the mall. Mother had struggled to make the ends meet. By the time she had gotten the belt together, sweat was running down her face.

"Whew! How does that feel?"

I could barely breathe. "Mother, it's too tight."

She wiped her face with the handkerchief she had pulled from her purse.

"I'll put an extra notch in it when we get home."

"Couldn't I go without the belt?"

"Absolutely not. It cuts your figure in half."

Now in my bedroom it was notched, so she could move to my face and hair.

"Did you put on enough hairspray?"

"Yes, Mother." If anyone ran into my hair, they'd probably lose an eye. It felt like strings of wire sticking out all over my head.

"How about the blush for your cheeks? You want to look healthy."

It sounded like I was on the auction block.

If I put on any more blush, I'd look like a freakin' clown, I thought to myself as Mother scanned me like an MRI.

"Do you have some freshening-up lipstick and powder in your purse?"

"Yes, I do. But I wish you had let me get the liquid face makeup. That powder makes me sneeze."

"Well, if you have to sneeze, get your hanky out right away and excuse yourself to go to the Ladies' Room."

This was starting to sound like a 50s coming-out debutante party instead of a high school dance.

"Now make sure you lightly touch his shoulder when you dance. Keep a little distance so he doesn't get the wrong idea."

Evidently, Mother had not watched television for quite a while. Dancing looked more like copulating while the entwined couples gyrated around the floor. I had seen a picture of snakes in a science magazine once that showed dozens of them twisting together as the males tried to hook up with the female. Teenagers dancing looked a lot like that on those music programs on TV.

"Okay, I guess we're ready." Mother made it sound like she had gotten her troops ready for battle and was sending them out.

As she dropped me off in front of the gym, she gave me one last look.

"Don't forget to smile, but don't show your teeth."

With that last admonition, she drove away. I was left in the social jungle by myself.

As the other parents dropped off their freshmen, I tried to look nonchalant as I sized up the competition from the girls and scoped out any interesting-looking boys. I was slightly disheartened by what I saw as available males. Boys don't catch up in height until their sophomore year. They all seemed short and gawky, except for the athletes. I heard that swimming was the best sport for developing every part of a guy's body. Maybe some freshmen swimmers would be coming.

The girls looked pretty much as I expected. Tiny tank tops, short skirts, and lots of eyeliner. You could tell which ones had been dressed by their mothers. They all looked like me.

As I waited my turn to show my school I.D. and pay my five-dollar entry fee, I glanced at the others in line around me. Most of the eyeliner girls were giggling and brazenly staring at the boys. The good-looking guys stared back and grinned, showing all their teeth. I noticed the line had become clumps of males and females gathered around each other. The boys were making lame jokes, and the short-skirted girls were obediently laughing.

"Excuse me, could you please move forward a little?" The line had stalled when the cheerleaders arrived. The boys were punching each other and rotating around them like a human carousel.

Wrong move on my part.

Several of them took the time to look me over.

"What's your hurry? They don't put out the cookies until later."

"Could that dress be any brighter? I'm going blind."

I clutched my purse next to my chest and lowered my head.

"Jeez, be careful with that hair. You could put somebody's eye out."

This came from a short boy in front of me who had turned to see what was happening behind him. He swiveled just as I lowered my head.

The gaggle of girls in back of me giggled and clutched the muscled arms of the athletes next to them. Obviously, the swim team had located the cheerleaders and vice versa.

When I got inside, I became aware that the lights hadn't been lowered yet.

Crap.

I stood out like a bright-blue glass bulb on a Christmas tree. I moved as quickly as I could so I could get to the Girls' Restroom to hide in one of the stalls until the music started. I had forgotten Mother's instructions about waiting outside until the dance music began.

When I went through the door, I could see the popular girls leaning forward towards the long mirror to apply more lipstick. They were eagerly discussing the boys.

"Did you see that one guy with the tight jeans?"

"Yeah, and he had a friend. This little dance may turn out interesting after all."

"It better. I bought this new outfit and don't want to waste it here."

I glanced at her clothes as I headed for one of the open stalls. Her outfit was barely there. She had the word "Princess" in sparkles on the tiny top she had stretched across her chest. Her skirt was thigh-level. Where were the clothes police at this dance? I hadn't noticed any teachers at the table at the entrance. It was manned by members of the student council who would get the profits. Probably to buy more eggs for their assemblies.

The girls finished and left. I strained to hear any music coming from the DJ at one end of the gym floor. After waiting for about ten minutes, I thought I'd take a look.

The blast of sound almost knocked me over. It was one of those songs that had a bass beat and muffled words from one of the current groups I'd hear on my bedroom radio at home. How could anybody dance to that?

As I watched the dancers, I noticed the girls' hips were inches away from the boys' crotches. Bumping and grinding must be the new dance steps. This was not going to be a one-two-three-four square series of turns with hands resting gently on the shoulders of their partners.

I saw some darker spots in the gym where some of the athletic equipment was stored. As I headed in their direction

I glanced surreptitiously at the moving bodies in front of the DJ. Since I wasn't paying attention to what was happening in front of me, I didn't realize someone was there until I literally bumped into him. He wasn't at eye level. I looked down and saw his belt buckle, so he wasn't short. I stepped back and saw all of him in one delighted glance. He was tall like a Greek god, and he had on a long-sleeved shirt and washed-out jeans. His hands were big, and one of them was grasping my arm.

"Sorry, excuse me, I didn't see you."

"No problem. Would you like to dance?"

I couldn't think of anything to say as he pulled me to the center of the floor.

Was this really happening? I must be in one of my alternate realities I create for myself where all is right with my world.

Maybe I looked attractive. Could that be possible with all the low-cut blouse girls in here?

The crowd seemed to be giving us some room. I tried to mimic what the other girls were doing. He was across from me, looking over my head. That didn't seem strange since dancers these days seldom looked in their partners' faces when they danced.

I must be doing pretty well. Dancers were backing away and watching us.

I tried to savor every moment as I threw myself into the music. I wished Mother could see me. I closed my eyes and luxuriated in the sensation. The music was loud, but I didn't care. My belt was digging into my waist, but I didn't feel anything. I was really dancing with one of the best-looking boys in the room. Maybe he saw the real me behind the weight. Maybe he wanted someone he could actually have an intelligent conversation with instead of the airheads he was probably used to. Maybe after this dance, he'd escort me to the snacks table to get something to drink and eat. We'd sit together on the metal folding chairs with our hands filled with small, cookie-filled napkins and soda. A slow dance would start. He'd take my hand. The other dancers would part as we reached the coveted spot in front of the DJ. I'd feel his arm encircling my waist. He'd pull me forward so my head rested on...

"Hey, watch where you're going, Chubs."

When I opened my eyes, I looked around in confusion. I was by myself, and other dancers were bumping into me.

"Where's your partner, Blue Bell?"

No, no, no. This is not happening.

I frantically surveyed the crowd. Where was he?

He didn't just leave me here, did he?

Then I saw him. He was laughing with several other boys grouped around him. He had a bunch of crumbled dollar bills in his hand. One of the blonde cheerleaders was whispering in his ear. He put his arm across her shoulders and they walked out the door. I was still standing where he had left me.

"You didn't think Jeff would actually dance with you." Some girl was shouting at me over the music.

"Wow, I think she really thought he was. What a dumb..."

I tried to get off the dance floor as fast as I could. I prayed that the heels I was wearing for the first time wouldn't make me fall.

I pushed through the bathroom door and hoped one of the stalls was available. I was having trouble seeing since hot tears were running rivulets down my cheeks.

Oh God, how could you do this to me? First the assembly and now this. It isn't fair.

I dug at my eyes with the small handkerchief Mother had placed in my purse. It soaked through in an instant. I sat down on the stool. Makeup was dropping from my chin onto my new dress.

I was used to sobbing quietly so as not to draw attention to myself to make matters worse if someone heard me.

I sat dejectedly in that stall for two hours until the dance ended. I had gotten the handicapped stall, so no one knocked on the door for me to hurry up.

A group of girls came in to fix their makeup or adjust their clothing at the close of the dance.

"God, what a boring dance. The only interesting thing was that fat girl dancing by herself."

"Did you hear what happened?"

"Something about the guys betting Jeff he wouldn't get the blue blimp on the dance floor."

"Jesus, how naïve could she be? Nobody like Jeff would give her a second look, much less dance with her."

The girls were giggling as they went out the door.

A bet. Of course, you stupid idiot. Why would someone who looked like him want to dance with you? This was just another scene from some teen movie where the homely girl gets taken in by the hot guy. My whole life is like a crappy teen film.

I waited another fifteen minutes so I was sure everyone had left.

My face and dress were a mess. I crept through the open door when the janitor had his back turned.

Mother's car was the only one waiting at the curb.

I got in and fastened my seat belt.

"What the hell happened? Look at your dress. I'll never get those stains out. Look at me when I'm talking to you."

"I don't want to talk about it."

I could feel her staring at me as she pulled away from the gym.

When we got home I rushed past my father up the stairs to my room. I locked myself in the bathroom and collapsed against the tub.

After about ten minutes I heard conversation outside the door.

"She doesn't want to talk about it. I have no idea what she did at the dance."

"Couldn't she make it at a freshmen dance, for crissakes?" My father was frustrated.

He jiggled the doorknob.

"She has it locked. Well, let's leave her alone for now."

"You know that dress is ruined. Maybe I can cut it down for her sister."

Their voices faded as they went back down the stairs.

We never did have that conversation about the dance. Mother took the dress into her room the next day. I guess they assumed I had ruined the evening for myself. I didn't want to look at their faces for several days. The disappointment hung in the air like dirty thoughts.

When I returned to school on Monday, it seemed everyone had forgotten about what had happened at the dance. I wasn't even a blip on their radar.

It was back to the small desks, the insensitive teachers, and the paper wads hitting me on the back of my neck in most of my classes.

Back to High School Hell

But as bad as it was in regular classes, it was like Dante's Inferno in P.E. The graduation requirements said that everyone had to have four years of physical education classes before they could graduate. Who thought that up? It was probably some fashionably thin mother on the School Board who had a cheerleader daughter. I couldn't win.

"You've got ten minutes to get out on the floor," the gym teacher yelled, as she locked the locker-room door. No desperate fatties could escape. To top off this horrendously hellish hour of my school day for four years, the P.E. outfit was approved by that snotty cheerleader's mother, who just knew her little darling would look so cute in this bright-yellow, one-piece, zippered gym suit with elastic in the legs. I still have the scars where that elastic cut into the upper part of my thighs.

"We're going to do warm-up aerobics with some strength tests a little later," the female drill sergeant said, as we lined up by height. Fat legs do not give someone height. I was in the front row, where the girls behind me could giggle at my barely contained cellulite jiggling all over the place as I jumped up and down for ten minutes.

Then it got even worse. You had to pull yourself over this high metal bar the two gym teachers held. Each teacher held an end. The non-fat girls used their arms to lift themselves over with no problems at all. Their slender legs followed like they were just meant to do that. If I had been a bodybuilder, I would have had the arm muscles to pull myself over that hateful elevated bar. As it was, I could pull up to my waist, but that was as far as I could get. My lower half stayed grounded. After several tries, while the girls behind me impatiently waited for their skinny turns, the gym teachers finally had to put a hand on each butt cheek and push me over, without getting hit in the face by the alarmed fat that was moving like chickens before their beheadings. I was mortified.

You'd think after fifty minutes of gym, I would be relieved to get back into the relative safety of the locker room. No such luck.

"Okay ladies, line up for your showers. Let's hurry now. You only have ten minutes to shower and get ready for your next class," the gym teachers said, as they stood by the entrance to the shower and watched as each naked girl went in. They told us it was to make sure that as girls came out, other girls could take their places.

Yeah, right.

They wanted to make sure no fat girls escaped into their clothes without a shower. It was part of their P.E. code or something. I hated it more than that rotten steel bar.

The shower room had white ceramic walls that made fat girls look like they were beached whales hung up against the white tiles. Barely any water came from the six nozzles.

One fat girl would take up one complete nozzle, which didn't endear her to the skinny girls waiting to shower quickly, so they had ample time to gossip and refurbish their makeup. As each girl came out, she was handed a washcloth-sized towel to dry off.

We had one girl in our class who was gaining weight in her stomach, but nowhere else. She disappeared one day. Those were the days when pregnant teens were sent away until they delivered. It was not accepted with such enthusiasm like today's high schools, where pregnant girls wear shirts with arrows pointing to their stomachs with slogans like "Under Construction," and can stay in school until their water breaks in History class.

Because of the horror I faced daily in my gym class, I thought seriously of getting pregnant to get out of it. But even the ugliest, most desperate high school boy doesn't want to have sex with a fat girl. No decent (thin) girl would want to date him in the future. So for the indecently fat girl, unless she wanted to pick up a dirty drunk in a dark alley, or the bald neighbor next door who was up for sex with anything, including a potted plant, getting pregnant was out as an option.

I did socialize sometimes. There were always the "pity" parties (the whole class had to be invited the parents would insist) and the car gropings. After all, I had a lot to grope, until the boy discovered that I didn't have as much on top as on the bottom. Then I'd get a look of disgust and "I got a test tomorrow, so I gotta get home to study." I would be unceremoniously dropped off on the sidewalk in front of my house. The "study for a test" would be an interesting excuse. Usually, the boys I got were seldom in school and when they were, it was for auto class.

There were times when I'd be invited to go to some girl's house to gossip, if I was standing right there when they decided to get together. I'd tell Mother when I got home. She'd get all excited, and we'd go out to get a new outfit. I had graduated from girdles to pantyhose. What a relief! My legs were no longer gouged by the girdle clasps, and I could breathe better. But even with shorts, I had to wear pantyhose. I was the only one in high school who wore pantyhose all the time, even in bed. Mother thought the constriction could possibly shrink the fat a little. It was uncomfortable but I had gotten used to being in some sort of clothing pain. I balked at wearing the super-sized pantyhose under my swimsuit, so I didn't go to the community pool anymore. Not a problem, since I had a suit that could probably be used as a life raft.

I remember the day Mother brought it into my room and laid it on my bed. It covered most of the bedspread. It was bright yellow and had skirts at the collar and waist.

"The skirts should help with the appearance. They cover some of the more pronounced areas on your figure. The color is cheerful, don't you think?"

Was she serious? I'd look like the sun coming up over the horizon. If I stepped into the water, the skirts would float around me like airplane blow-up life preservers.

Nope, no swimming again this summer.

Summer was far away. I had something wonderful in the here and now. I was breathless with anticipation. Waiting for the doorbell to ring, I sat carefully on the edge of the bed in my brand new clothes. Mother had splurged, and we had gone to an up-scale store to find a nice shirt-and-shorts set for this special occasion.

Often, I got up to go to the window. I pulled the curtain aside a bit, so I could look out to see if the girls were coming down the walk, or getting out of their mothers' cars to come up to the front door to ring the bell or knock. When the agreed-upon hour would arrive, I'd be ready to answer the bell. As the minutes clicked away, I made up excuses why they were late. They needed more time for putting on their makeup, or someone to drive them. They were involved in a minor fender-bender and were stuck at the accident scene, or perhaps they weren't sure of the address, but had misplaced my telephone number.

I sat motionless on the edge of my bed for an hour. I listened for the door or telephone.

Of course, they never came. I would hear mother slowing climbing the stairs to knock on my door.

"Are you sure that was the right time? Maybe they got the wrong house. Do they have the telephone number?"

I had stopped hearing her plaintive voice. She stood at the door for a little while, then turned and went back downstairs. I could imagine the disappointment on her face.

Later, I'd hear her talk to my father. They would speak in low voices. At times, my father would forget to keep his voice down.

"Why doesn't she have any friends?"

Mother murmured a reply.

I had gotten under the covers in my bed, after changing my clothes and putting the new ones in my bottom drawer. I cried quietly for hours.

The next day at school, I hoped the girls would come over to tell me why they hadn't come. When I saw them and smiled, they looked past me as if I wasn't there. Then I realized they had been only being civil. I'm sure they didn't remember inviting me. I was an irritating presence, an afterthought in their lives.

For my sophomore and junior years in high school, I stayed to myself. I'd slink along close to the wall when going to my classes. I would make sure I got there in plenty of time, so I could hunch down in my desk as much as possible. I would press forcefully into the desk bar until it really hurt, so I didn't hang over so much.

Some of the fat girls found a way to let themselves know they were alive. Several of them were "cutters." They'd slice open their arms with whatever was handy – a pulled-apart paperclip, a mechanical pencil with the lead broken off, and a knife from home in their purses or backpacks they could take out and use in the stalls in the bathrooms.

Most people couldn't tell, but I knew the signs of deep depression that led them to mutilate themselves over and over. Long sleeves all year, bloody toilet paper in the hand-towel bins, seepage on the class chairs.

I guess they had their own little clique, too. I heard they exchanged information about where to cut and how to do it, so there wasn't a lot of blood that could get them noticed. The Internet was a terrific resource. Lots of advice for depressed fat-girl cutters. Photos, too, so you could understand, if you were a fat-girl visual learner.

When I started to lose weight through bulimia, I was especially judgmental, like a former smoker or a recovering drug addict. They didn't have to stay fat. They could do something about it. The cutting was gross. They were already fat. Now they were mutilated for life AND fat!

Chapter 4

Salvation

One day during my senior year, I went to the Girls' bathroom before my first morning class. All the stalls were taken. Guess I'd have to go between classes. Then I heard them – the sounds that would change my life forever. I heard vomiting sounds coming from each separate cubicle, and they were in sync. What the hell?

Finally, the doors all unlatched at the same time. The popular skinny girls came out, wiping the corners of their bow-shaped mouths with the tips of their salon fingernails. They rinsed out their mouths with little bottles of mouthwash they had. Exchanging amused glances, they followed each other out. I could hear them outside the door, laughing and making comments about what they would throw up for lunch.

After my first class, I asked a couple of fat girls what was going on. They said the girls were bulimics who made a party out of eating together, and then vomiting as a group in the bathrooms.

"You mean they aren't all born like that? Some of them could be overweight if they didn't vomit up everything?"

The fat girls were skeptical.

"They probably were born skinny, but want to be thinner or stay that way, so they throw up everything they eat so they can eat more. It's gross."

I couldn't tell whether they thought it was distasteful because the girls were throwing up what fat girls treasured the most – food – or they thought, "Well, we may be fat but we don't do that," kind of gross.

I didn't care one way or the other. I was overjoyed. It was like how I pictured my first orgasm would feel. I didn't have to be fat. Even my fat legs and butt could be reduced to empty skin if I didn't let any calories get to them. I had gotten an A+ in Health class. I knew about calories. I just thought we were stuck with them, and had to work them off with years of gym. Not something I was willing to do. After high school, I never wanted to see a girls' locker room or a nude girl again as long as I lived.

What a revelation! Why hadn't Mother told me about this magnificent secret way to lose weight and stay thin?

"Mother, do you know some girls have vomiting parties in the Girls' bathrooms at school?"

Mother was aghast.

"That's just awful. What would those girls' mothers say if they knew their daughters were doing something so dangerous to their bodies like that?'

I found out later their mothers were bulimics, too. I guess Mother was behind the times. Being dead was better than being fat. They knew that, and I certainly knew it. We usually had at least one fat-girl suicide each year. Everyone kind of expected that one of us would just not return to school, either because we had gotten fatter over the summer and had moved to a different school, or killed ourselves because "who'd want to live, if they were going to be fat forever."

The fat-girl scenario about Internet death wouldn't ever apply to me, though. I knew the Internet could turn on a fat girl as well as be her anonymous best friend. The recent story about a homely, fat girl (synonymous terms in the thin world) who hanged herself because a boy who didn't exist sent her one last email that was horrendously awful, is common in our world. The mother of a thin did her in. Fascinating level of cruelty. It was just another arena for us to be butchered in. Fat girls are constantly being deceived on the Internet. You'd think they would pay attention when one of them does herself in. But since they always crave affection, they'll choose to believe anything and rationalize any behavior.

The processing of the fat-girl Internet death by our very own high school elite lent a whole new meaning to casual conversation about getting rid of the visible fat-stain in their midst. They didn't bother keeping their voices down as they cruised the high school hallways. After all, school was for learning. They had found the fat-girl death-by-Internet both entertaining and instructive.

"Why would they prosecute the mother who set up the fake boyfriend for that fat slob?"

"Yeah, she was doing the right thing. What happened to justice in our society?"

"Too bad there weren't pictures. Bet the rope had to be several feet thick to hold her up until her neck snapped."

"Probably couldn't find the rope around her neck to cut her down with all that flab in the way."

They laughed.

"Good one."

If this was good, discussing their own reign of terror on a fat girl they knew was deliciously better.

We found out later they had decided to do the same thing to a fat girl from our high school. She eventually hanged herself in her closet, after our high school popular clique had located her on her website, and begun a relentless campaign to destroy her. Vicious emails, pornographic pictures of fat girls being assaulted, and finally daily messages telling her she should kill herself to do the world a favor. It was fun for them. One less disgusting fat girl in the world. Deleted from the gene pool. A real public service.

"I loved the emails Chelsea sent to our own fat nightmare."

"The part about her being the last girl on earth, and even then he wouldn't date her was so great."

"Man, she was so easy to convince. Must have been really desperate."

"What fatass isn't?"

After they had cut her down, the police found the last nasty emails Chelsea had sent. The suicidal fat girl had left them up on the screen. The emails got on YouTube faster than a skinny girl could say, "Awesome!" when she saw them. It was the talk of the school for a while. No one was ever held responsible. We fat girls knew. We always knew who despised us the most at school. But we faded into the shadows rather than face the brutality that was sure to come if we accused them.

Perfecting My Technique

For the rest of my senior year in high school, I had my own little vomiting parties whenever I ate. And I ate anything I wanted; usually chips, candy, and mini-cakes. I'd hide them in my backpack in my locker. At lunch, I'd retrieve them, and eat everything in the handicapped stall in the Girls' bathroom. It had the most room for my various piles of food. The toilet was quite a distance from the stall door, since wheelchairs had to be rolled in. That extra space was just what I needed. Anyone coming in wouldn't be able to see what I had in there. Most kids didn't go near the handicapped stall, anyway. If the hall monitors ducked in to check on the bathrooms and found you in the handicapped stall, they waited for you to come out. Since you probably weren't handicapped, you'd be sent to the Principal's Office. There were federal laws and all.

This was 'way beyond wonderful. I could eat as much as I wanted, throw it back up, and load up again. Miracle of miracles!

I had to learn on my own how to do it so nobody could find out. Fortunately, the Internet had loads of sites where I could get advice, and step-by-step instructions on how to be bulimic. The biggest websites were devoted to college-age girls, so I knew I would have plenty of company at the university. Maybe I could pick up some extra bulimic tips from all my new eating-disordered compatriots in the hundreds of chat rooms they had going.

I decided I would design my lifestyle around my bulimia. Instead of focusing on food as an enemy, I could welcome it as my best pal. This was easy for a perfectionist like me. My OCD really worked for me here. I was smart and had a usable mental disorder. I figured Mother had given me these traits along with her heavy legs. Finally, something positive about having a dysfunctional parent. This was going to work out just fine.

One of the first things I learned was not to gorge at meals, either at home or in public. Of course, it played nicely into the bulimic program, because fat girls were not expected to overeat when they were with family or friends. They were unappetizing enough to look at as it was. It would be downright beyond disgusting to watch them put shovelfuls of food in their maws, and watch them swallow without chewing. They would resemble sea lions that sit around all day, snacking on spawning fish. In fact, there were rumors that the sea lion population would have to be culled to save the ovulating fish. A sea-lion shooting fest was on the legislative menu.

"Damn," said the slender majority, "why couldn't they do the same with fat girls? Just thin their population by making them disappear."

Oh wait. People were already doing that to the best of their abilities.

Fat girls lived on the periphery of society. They wouldn't dare think of putting one of their fat feet over the established social-thinness line. They were aberrations.

Hide the chips and dip if you see a fat girl waddle through the door. Make sure she pays the bill if you deign to eat with her, as she probably ordered the most food, anyway. Don't be seen talking with her, unless you have to. If the fat slob was blocking the movie screen, a person had the right to loudly demand:

"Could you move? The rest of us would like to see the movie, too."

Actually, I executed a strategic plan when I went alone to the movies.

I sat in the back of movie theatres, with my food cache hidden in my huge purse. I knew I couldn't get in the food line. The ridicule would be unending. I would stock up before I went. I was careful to choose food that didn't make any sound. My bags of candy had to be emptied out and unwrapped, before putting them in plastic bags tucked quietly away. I would unscrew the tops of the glass soda bottles, so they wouldn't make any noise when I opened them. Cans were out of the question – a dead giveaway. Heads would turn.

"She had to bring her own supply. How disgusting!"

Nobody stays quiet when a fat girl eats. People sanctimoniously "for-your-own-good" pontificate on the benefits of healthy eating when they see a fat girl put food in her mouth. They don't even have to be family; anyone can harass a fat girl. She's a walking target, the last to be discriminated against. Who the hell wants that?

The Good Life

I could get people to love me, and eat all I wanted. It was a great world! I ate at all hours of the day. Secretly, of course, so as not to draw attention. I shopped at different stores at various times of the day. I had hiding places in my room and in my book bag. I couldn't store food in my locker. They were too close together. Anyone would look in my locker when I opened it as if they had the right. Fat girls had no privacy. After all, they were fat, so they obviously didn't care what people did or thought around them. You had to earn the right to say "no" to others. Fat girls hadn't earned it. They were up for grabs anytime and anywhere for humiliation. Sometimes, boys who couldn't get noticed by any girls would paw at fat girls as they walked by in the hallways. They would purposely bump into them in the classroom doorways, so the fat girl looked like she was struggling to fit through the door.

There was one hallway fat girls particularly avoided, even if they had to go outside and around the building to get into their classes. The popular girls called it "The Perfect 10 Hallway," because they could walk it like models while the boys, lined up on each side, made admiring comments and yelled out "10s" while the girls pranced by. If a fat girl late for class for any reason (crying in the restroom, pulling her girdle down so it didn't ride up her thighs, eating alone in the handicapped stall, for instance), and she had to walk through the gauntlet to get to her next class, it was a horror show.

She would lower her head, wrap her oversized sweater around her, and walk as quickly as she could through the groups of jeering adolescent males.

"Man, she has to be a minus 10. Look at those legs."

"Yeah, cannibals could live off those for a month!"

The laughter could be heard in the surrounding classrooms. Kids would peer through the doors at the spectacle. It was like the Roman Coliseum, and all the thumbs were down for death. Only this was a "living death." At least, the Christians were eventually torn to pieces by the lions. The "high school lions" here hollered, pounced, and grabbed, but didn't end the torture until the fat girl made it to the end of the hallway, and sobbing, stumbled into the nearest empty classroom. I heard what happened in that dreadful hallway for people like me. After that, even though it killed me to be late to class, I would risk it rather than pass through that brutal human gauntlet.

The boy at the head of the hallway would catch sight of a fat girl heading hurriedly their way. He would holler to the other cretins standing on both sides:

"Hey, we got a live one!"

"Hey baby, how many people you got under those clothes?" The lout would grab her skirt and jiggle it as if to see if bodies would roll out. The other watching pieces of human crap would yell and slap one another. It was probably the most they concentrated on school all day.

Several of the pimply gawky males who were often the targets of the other boys, now had their chance to be a part of the exclusive male crowd. They were especially vicious as their victim tried to run by. Pulling at her breasts, trying to get their unwashed hands under her skirt, they were like creatures in the dark with a million appendages ready to grope and hurt. The fat girl would put her books against her chest like some sort of desperate shield.

"C'mon, Tubbo, give it up." Their fists full of clothing would make buttons pop off or zippers rip. At this point, their prey would scream and draw the attention of a teacher in one of the classrooms. The teacher didn't actually come out, but would yell from behind the door:

"Okay, that's enough. Get to class or you'll all get detention."

Since many of the abusers were football players, and detention meant being late to practice, they would leave, nonchalantly shoving the fat girl as they sauntered by. She would be left by herself, her books scattered at her feet, her clothes disheveled, her face tear-streaked. Nobody helped her. She didn't expect it. She would lean over carefully, holding her blouse together with one hand, while she picked up her school folders and books with the other. She'd be too upset to go to class. She'd tell the School Nurse that she had a migraine and needed to go home.

Such a charmingly crude high school ritual. A scene out of any realistic teenage movie at an American high school. Forgotten in an instant by the perpetrators; forever embedded in the fat girl's mind. Yes, we had to make accommodations wherever we went to survive, including at the local movie theatre.

How I longed to put one leg over the other while I was sitting in a desk or a theatre seat instead of crossing them at my fat ankles. Pushing my side into the bar on the desk chair gave me a perpetual red slash resembling a long knife cut.

I didn't eat in the school cafeteria. For one thing, the metal chairs were attached to the tables so you had to slide in. Half of me would be hanging off the chair if I tried. I would walk home for lunch, since we didn't live far from the high school. I would have a peanut-butter-and-jelly sandwich, a bowl of soup, and a soda everyday. My daily lunch probably contained around 3,000 calories for the first three years of high school. On the way back, I would scarf down a couple of chocolate bars I had hidden in my backpack.

When I joyfully became bulimic the last half of my senior year, I didn't go home for lunch. I found a maintenance shed behind the hated gym and binged on what I had zippered up in my backpack the day before. I crammed in as much junk food as I could. I had to be careful the zipper didn't go off its tracks, or I'd have to ask Mother for a new backpack. I could just hear the conversation we'd have.

I would try to get her after she had a few fridge drinks, so she was relaxed and unwary.

"Mother, I need to go to the store to get a new backpack." I'd be sitting next to her on the couch, but on the edge, so I could move fast if I needed to.

She'd look up with her already red-rimmed eyes with their bleary off-in-the-distance gaze.

"What happened to the one I just got you?"

"I tried to jam too many books in it. The zipper broke." My voice would be a monotone, but my hands would be gripped together to keep them from shaking. Dialogues with Mother were to be avoided whenever possible. I seldom came out on the winning end.

She'd look for it behind my back, as if I always had it on whenever she'd see me. Her hand jerkily moved towards me.

"Lemme see it."

"I had to throw it out. I'm sorry. I know it was a lot of money."

"Damn right. Do you think money grows on trees?"

If money grew on trees, I would've found the nearest one and taken off long ago, I thought wryly.

"I'll be real careful with the new one, Mother. I'll get a bigger one this time. I have a lot of heavy books from the advanced classes I'm taking."

Maybe she'd notice "the advanced classes" bit, and I would be complimented on how hard I worked in school and how proud of me she was.

What dream world are you living in, I thought regretfully, as I eluded her hand reaching for the non-existent backpack.

"What did you say?" She hadn't heard a thing for the last several minutes. Her eyes were half-closed, as she began to slump back onto the pillows at the end of the couch. I had to get her before she went to sleep.

"Mother, I'm just going to get a few dollars from your wallet, so I can get a new book bag in that store near school when I finish my classes for the day. Is that okay?"

I'd hear a mumble as she fell back. I'd put her feet up. I'd hope it was payday, so she wouldn't notice any money missing, since I was sure she wouldn't remember our conversation. That day after school, I'd get one that was exactly like the one she bought me.

No, this was a fantasy scenario I didn't want to happen.

I was absolutely sure how much junk food I could cram in.

No broken zippers here, I thought smugly, as I wolfed down the backpack's secret contents.

It took about twenty minutes to voraciously eat about five pounds of food. When my stomach hurt, I'd stop. I saved the last ten minutes of the lunch period for throwing it all back up.

I had a routine I had established that worked perfectly for the time I had for lunch.

When I couldn't eat any more without grabbing my middle in pain, I started my purging routine in the maintenance shed. I always jammed something under the doorknob when I was safely inside, just in case the yard guy came by for his rake or shovel. I figured he'd jiggle the knob for a bit, and then go off and do something else. At least, that was how I imagined it would happen in the worst-case scenario when someone would try to open the door.

Anyway, I was pretty fast with my ritual. I could probably get out of there if I had to, before the person came back. I had everything down to the minute. First, I pulled the hair behind my ears. Then I took out a tall kitchen garbage bag, opened it, and using my right hand, I put two fingers as far down my throat as I could get them until I gagged. To get the food coming back up, I'd think of the most horrible mental images I could create to make me want to retch. A Styrofoam cup full of maggots crawling through snot and excrement was one that worked really well in a time crunch. The chunks of food would come up fast. I'd keep doing it until I could taste the stomach bile in my mouth.

Out would come the mouthwash to disguise the smell and hand wipes to repair any makeup that got damaged while I was vomiting. I didn't want pieces of sponge cakes stuck on my chin. I had learned my lesson about some foods, like peanut butter, that wouldn't willingly come up as easily. I'd have to stand up, so the gobs could clear the esophagus. Bending over from a crouched position didn't work for gummy stuff. I saved the "hard-to-vomit-in-a-hurry" items for home purging, when I could take my time.

Pretty soon I could eat, vomit, clean up, fix my makeup, and be in class early. I would get the maggot image in my mind before bending over. My gagging fingers didn't even have to go back too far into my throat before everything started on its way back up.

I liked the tall kitchen garbage bags, because they had those red elastic hoops that pulled together to close the bag. I could put it in my oversized backpack, and casually drop it into the garbage can near the back door of the locker rooms. Of course, I had strategically planned how to dispose of it, as well as how to do it before I first tried.

I had to be careful in the afternoon classes, because I had nothing in my stomach. I couldn't always depend on the teacher lecturing, or the students talking to cover the sounds. I would have a pen or pencil handy to repetitiously tap on the top of the desk, until my stomach gurgling stopped. If it were really loud, I'd have to take desperate measures and drop a book or rustle my papers vigorously. Sometimes, I couldn't get to it in time, and the noise would be heard by those seated around me. They'd look at each other, and often say something mean out loud.

"Man, you'd think she'd fill up enough at lunch. Maybe she has to eat every hour. Must be a bottomless pit."

"Can you keep it down? I'm trying to learn here."

This one came from a boy who spent most of his time throwing paper wads at the dummy across the room.

I was a distraction from the boredom of the class. It was just another day in the life of a high school fat girl.

Well, I was going to be skinny. They would always be dumbasses. It was little consolation, though, when I was mistreated.

I had something they didn't. I had a secret none of them would ever know. And I was the absolute best at what I was doing.

I knew I was the champion bulimic at school. I deserved some kind of award with Best Campus Bulimic written in fancy font across it. What a ceremony that would be. The band would play, the rich kids (usually the cheerleaders and football players) would clap, Mother would dab at her eyes with pride, the principal would hand me this gigantic trophy my father would beamingly hold for me, and I'd wave to all, with a somewhat queenly hand movement. After the ceremony, the bathroom-purge beauties would rush to congratulate me.

I jest. I do that a lot.

Well, at least I didn't upchuck in groups or in bathrooms others used, where I could get caught. Of course, the worse that could happen to the thins was that they lied, and said they had an upset stomach from worrying about a test or something. The ignorant staff would believe anything you told them if you were pretty. I didn't have that luxury. The thin girls really didn't care if you knew what they were doing, anyway. It was part of being cool. Only the truly popular girls were invited to join the bathroom-vomiting cliques.

I was above them, superior in every way. But my triumph had to be kept secret. It was enough for me, since I was losing weight. Some of the mid-level popular kids were starting to talk to me now. I was in.

My fat friends fell away like grain sacks rolling down a hill. I didn't need them anymore, now that my weight was coming down. I cruelly ignored them, like the thin girls did. I didn't want to be associated with them. I had non-fat people who talked to me now.

I heard the best words in the English language for the first time: "Have you lost weight? You look really good." Every time I heard that, I would promise myself to lose more weight. I had to hear it over and over again. It was literally life to me.

Home Life

My home-bulimic routine was solid. No one came in my room, so my bathroom was mine alone. Since Mother sometimes poked her head in and looked around while she was cleaning upstairs, I had to be careful about food left in plain sight. I had a tall bookcase with recessed shelves that were perfect for storing bags of cheese balls and chocolate drops, my staples. Under my clothes in my chest-of-drawers, I would lay out my larger chocolate bars. They were flat, even the extra-large ones, and so there were no suspicious bulges. I had to watch how many I'd stack on top of one another, or my drawer wouldn't close.

The only chocolate I didn't like was dark, the one supposedly good for you. My favorites were the round peanut butter, chocolate patties that came four to a flat package. I kept the temperature in my room at around 65 degrees. It got a little chilly in winter, but keeping the chocolate from melting was my primary concern. As I lost body fat, though, I had to turn it up several degrees, or my shivering would disrupt my eating.

Soft food that lasted for months was a real find. Usually, it came in easy-to-unwrap packages, so I didn't make much noise when I opened them. I had to sacrifice ice cream products when I binged, because I had no way to keep them cold. And it wasn't like I could traipse downstairs, grab a half-gallon, run back to my room and shove it down before it melted. It might be missed, too, or become too messy to work with.

I was the perfect food addict. I was highly organized, loved my addiction, and knew I'd never give it up. Sitting on the floor, I was in the middle of an island of delicious tidbits in various-colored packaging. Before I started my methodical bingeing, I would regard my products with lustful anticipation. Bags of chips went in the mound to my left, and sacks of candy in stacks on my right. To the back of me, I had bottles of cola to wash everything down with. I ate everything in one binge, so I didn't have to worry about expiration dates on the packages. I also had scissors, so I could cut off the tops of the bags to expedite things. The individual pieces of candy were removed from the bags and the covers peeled off, so I wouldn't be slowed down by having to unwrap them separately.

The candy kisses were a challenge, unless I had the forethought to set them free from their foil papers before I consumed them. Unwrapping each chocolate-shaped kiss, I had to watch carefully for the little pull paper at the top of each one. Often, it would not come all the way out, unless I gently coaxed it away from the spherical treat. Otherwise, I'd pop it in my mouth, and taste the paper mixed with the chocolate. It would take precious eating time, and be pretty messy getting the paper out from the chocolate coating my mouth.

Planning was everything. I got really fast at candy peeling. One of my edible tricks would involve "crusty cheese-ball fingers" and soft chocolate. Eating a lot of fried cheese balls coats your fingers with orange crusts. Rather than lick the crust away and then pick up a chocolate, I would let the sticky buildup on my fingers become attached to the candy kiss or other chocolate drop when I reached into the candy pile. It was a great combination, and got rid of the leavings on my fingers without my stopping to wipe them off, or lick them clean. Imaginative, tasty, and quick. I was truly a genius in binge-eating techniques.

I could probably write a best-seller about how to binge eat, I thought gleefully.

My large throw rug was rolled halfway in front of me, in case I needed to cover everything fast. I didn't anticipate any visitors, since no one paid any particular attention to me at home, either. My sister was the thin pretty one that my parents seemed to thrive on. The five-year age gap kept me from being interested in what she was doing. Anyway, she got all the attention she needed. My parents usually went their own separate ways now, and met up for dinner once in a while.

I loved fast food, but since I didn't have a car, I couldn't hit the distant fast-food places. That was troublesome, too, because if a restaurant was in walking distance from my home, there might be students from the high school or neighbors who were eating there. Fat girl in a fast-food place – perfect fodder for gossip, on-the-spot humiliation and reports back to my parents, who thought I was on an eternal diet. I could imagine the embarrassing scene. Nosy neighbors would corner me as I sat down to eat.

"Are you sure you want to eat that? I know your parents are concerned about you. I can show you the calorie count for those."

The high school crowd would have some entertainment with their meals.

"Hey fatcheeks, I've got a little cheeseburger left."

"Thunderthighs, I've got a few French fries here, if you wanna come get 'em."

"Here piggy, piggy." Originality was not one of their strong points. In fact, I.Q.s of titmice were more their aptitudes.

I didn't totally have to give up fast food. When Mother dropped me off at our local warehouse-shaped store, I was the happiest fat girl around. I wouldn't waste time shopping. It would be humiliating, since I had to try on what I was going to buy. The clothes were so humongous, they usually cost more. I'd rather spend the money elsewhere.

And I learned my lesson about clothes-buying the first time Mother let me shop for myself there. They had a low-paid, middle-aged woman in an ugly blue jacket posted in front of the dressing rooms. You had to show her what you were taking in. She handed you a plastic number corresponding to the number of items you wanted to try on. Since the store only allowed three at a time, this poverty-wage loser would count the clothes by pawing through them. Since I had such large sizes, it was hard to tell how many items I had. There was so much material. This dressing-room door guard would hold up each piece of clothing I had over my arm, to see where one ended and the other began. She wouldn't take my word for it. Then this cretin would wave the pair of jeans or shirt, like a sail on a sailboat in a regatta. She would loudly announce, "One pair of jeans. I could swear it looked like two," or "These big blouses get tangled."

I stood there like a stricken sow, waiting for the slaughterhouse hammer to come down. Mutely mortified, I looked at the floor until she was finished. Rather than get my plastic number, I muttered something and walked away as fast as I could. To add insult to injury, she yelled for the whole store to hear, "Hey, don't you want to try these on? Okay, I'll put them back on the Maxi rack."

That was the first and last time I looked at clothes to buy there. It was hard to move through the shelves and racks, anyway. They were so crowded, I'd knock at least five or six items off with my hips, or the hanging flab on my arms, before I could get to the section I needed.

You may think I don't like our local huge box-shaped store after such an awful experience. I LOVED that store. It had a fast-food franchise. It was fast-food heaven.

On subsequent trips, I'd head right for the fast-food restaurant when I entered the store. It was located near the exit, too. Perfect.

As I stood in line to order, I played out a scene that would have impressed any drama teacher. I'd keep craning my neck, as if I was waiting for someone to join me. When I got to the counter, I'd say in a loud voice, "Well, I'll go ahead and order for both of us." I'd pick up several hamburger combos and several of their apple pies. I'd ask the counter person to put each combo in a separate bag, with an apple pie in each. I put one large drink cup inside the other one. I'd carry the bags and cup to the soda stand. I filled it with several kinds of soda. I would look around to scope out the seating and the other eaters. If there were young kids there, I'd leave. Kids had no problem announcing to the world, "Momma, that fat lady has two bags. Why does she have two bags for just her?" I'd escape through the exit doors, before I heard the parent respond.

If there weren't any children, the place wasn't crowded, and there were empty booths at the back, sometimes I'd take a chance and sit in one of the booths near the restrooms. Most people didn't like to sit in those booths.

If there weren't any booths at the back of the small eating area, I'd get the food to go. I'd find a space between parked cars at the far end of the lot, and rapidly eat. I'd feel like that guy who won that yearly hotdog contest. I'd take a big bite of my hamburger, and then gulp some soda. I'd wait for the soda to turn the hamburger in my mouth to mush before I swallowed it.

If I decided to eat in the restaurant, I'd put one of the combos on the other side of the table, so it appeared to be two people eating instead of just me. I'd finish one combo, then look around several times to see if anyone was watching me. If I were safe, I'd slide my combo sack with its wrappings, off the table to the bench part of the seat closest to the window or wall.   I crushed the bag as small as I could make it. I'd pick it up, then get up, as if I needed to refill my drink. I'd hold the crushed bag under my arm. There was plenty of fat to cover it. As I made my way to the soda station, I dropped the bag into the closest trash receptacle. I'd take out the cup inside the other one when no one was paying attention. I had my back to the patrons. I would wait until the soda station was clear before I approached. I filled this new one with soda. It looked as if I had only the one container.   I would make my way back to the booth, and sit on the side where the other untouched combo was waiting. It looked as if I had just sat down to eat my meal. I'd then finish off the second combo. When I finished, I'd put the empty wrappers in the bag, close it securely, and put it in the bin next to the restrooms at the back of the store.

Now it was time to get rid of the food. When I went in the Women's restroom, I'd head for my favorite stall, the one for the handicapped. Like the one at school, it was roomy and the toilet was set far back from the door.   No one could see my feet as I vomited standing up. The floors were dirty, so I didn't want to go down on my knees. I'd bend my head, start my fingers down my throat, and as if on cue, the combos and apple pies would be on their way back up. I'd flush the toilet several times to mask the sounds of my retching, and to get rid of the large chunks of food landing in the bowl.

This entire process – eating, vomiting, and cleaning myself up - would take around 45 minutes, if there wasn't a line in front of the counter, and a booth was available towards the back. If I had any extra time before Mother picked me up, I'd go back to the counter, and buy six of their chocolate chip cookies for later. I'd wrap them in napkins, and hide them in one of the zippered pouches in my backpack. There was plenty of room for them, because I emptied out the books and any food left from my school binge in my bedroom before we'd go to the store. I'd make sure the food was securely hidden.

I always did a room check before I closed my door. No food wrappers could be showing anywhere.

I had my backpack with me wherever I went. I wore a backpack because Mother said it made me look intelligent. I think she thought it would hide my neck and back fat. I had kept my hair longer to cover as much of my face and neck as I could. But if the wind were blowing, Mother would try to pat any wind-blown hair back into place before others could see the fleshy bulges when we appeared in public. Before I opened the car door at our humongous box store, Mother would have some parting comments:

"Do you have your brush with you? I'd like to work on your bangs, and smooth down your hair a bit. I've got some light lipstick that will blend in with the color of your face."

Red lipstick would draw attention to it. We couldn't have that.

Mother would give me an hour, and then be waiting for me outside the entrance.

"Did you find anything to wear?"

"They were out of sizes 22s and 24s."

Mother would heave one of her enormous "I've-got-a-fat-daughter" sighs, murmur, "God give me strength" under her breath, and we'd head for home.

I should mention that another reason for regurgitating before I rode home with Mother was her stomach-churning driving technique.

My grandfather had taught my mother to drive when she was sixteen, so she could get back to the store faster when school let out. Knowing the abject fear Mother had of her father, it was a traumatic experience for her, and had terrible lasting effects on how she drove.

It was one of Mother's bedtime stories.

"My father had no patience with me. If he wasn't criticizing everything I did in the car, he was looking at me in disdain when I did something stupid because I was so nervous. I was never fast enough off the brake to the accelerator with one foot, so to save time and so he wouldn't say something mean, I'd use both feet to drive. Of course that made things a little jerky, but it was the only way I could do it fast enough to satisfy him. He never looked at my fat legs, so he didn't notice that I was using both of my feet."

Sometimes from under the bedcovers, I'd hazard a question.

"Mother, couldn't your stepmother teach you?"

Her face took on a sad expression. In a resigned voice, she said, "She wasn't allowed to learn to drive. My father said she didn't need to go anywhere anyhow, and if she went somewhere, it would be with him. So she never learned and couldn't teach me."

Mother paused for a moment as if something had just occurred to her.

"You know, I bet she didn't like going in a car anyway, because your grandfather was sometimes drunk when he drove. That must have scared her to death."

So, driving with Mother was a really unpleasant experience. The car would stop and go with such erratic movements that I usually felt like throwing up in the car, even on short distances. It was definitely a good thing I didn't have anything in my stomach.

When we'd finally get home, in addition to feeling nauseated, if my father was home, he'd remark when we came in without any shopping bags:

"Couldn't find anything again? Maybe you should look in those stores that have extra sizes for big girls."

Terrific.

On the way upstairs to my room, I'd hear them in the kitchen, talking in muted tones about another fruitless shopping attempt to find me something to wear.

"She's got to have something new. Her shirts and pants are coming apart."

"Don't they have stores for overweight girls?"

"She's more than overweight. When I'm with her, we go right to the Plus sizes in the women's sections. It's so frustrating. All these cute outfits for girls her age."

"Well, if she'd quit eating us out of house and home, maybe she'd lose some pounds. Do you know if I'm coming downstairs and she's going upstairs, one of us has to lean against the wall or banister sideways, so one of us can go up or down? It's ridiculous the way she looks."

"That's just the thing. I make sure I buy nutritious food when I shop. I don't buy junk food at all because it would be such a temptation for her. I make her clean her plate, but she doesn't ask for seconds, and all the things I make are good for her. Maybe it's something physical. I read this article about metabolism."

"She's a teenager! They have the fastest metabolism of any of us."

"Then it's probably my fat legs. It's probably my fault the way she is."

"That doesn't excuse her fat everywhere else. It's 'Take Your Daughter to Work Day" tomorrow. The guys I work with don't even know I have an older daughter at home. How could I explain her? It would be embarrassing for all of us, her included."

I'd stop on the stairs, so I could hear if either one of them would defend me, or say something about my feelings, or that "they loved me anyway." Didn't happen.

Once I got to my room, I'd close the door quietly so they wouldn't know I had been listening. Then it was emotional feeding time. I'd grab all kinds of junk food from whatever hiding places were in my immediate reach, and pour them on the floor in one big pile. No careful planning or organizing the binges these times. I could hear they didn't like me, much less love me. I was a constant embarrassment, a frustrating lump of a girl who didn't care about her appearance. Someone even her parents didn't love. A pariah at school and at home. I was a fat girl. My sister could get away with anything because she was thin. I didn't get away with anything because I was abnormally fat. Not leftover baby fat. My fat was glaringly grotesque.

It was worse than having some terrible disease. Most diseases could be cured. They had inoculations to keep people from getting diseases. There was no shot for fat girls. They were lazy slobs who chose to stuff their faces and grow as big as a house. It would have been better if I'd had some incurable illness. I'd get some sympathy and compassion for how I looked. To the outside world of the thins, I was the ultimate ugliness. I was fat.

My parents would frequently have these conversations. I was never included. I didn't exist as a person for them, either. As Shakespeare would say, "The unkindest cut of all."

After I was satiated from my frenzied emotional binge, and had gotten rid of the evidence with my toilet ritual, I'd lie on my bed and fantasize about what it would be like to have my own car.

I would spend as little time as possible at home. They wouldn't have to look at me with such disappointment, with such pitiless anger, with such total frustration, with such damning blame. They'd go on to talk about other things, like money, their jobs, their plans, just like a family without a fat girl as a daughter.

My dream car would give me so much freedom to get my food fixes. It would be heaven to go through the drive-thru and load up. I would close my eyes and imagine eating while driving, stopping and eating in the car, or going to a park where I could sit at a picnic table and gorge. I could go to stores out of my neighborhood to get my junk food supplies. I could put them in the locked trunk, until I could sneak down after dark, and bring them up to my bedroom. It was blissful just thinking about the possibilities.

Home Life – Part 2

When I wasn't frantically eating to salve the hurt from the latest parent discussion about me, my regular bingeing was something truly to be admired. My brilliant eating-disorder ritual was the epitome of bulimic design and execution. I was like a general organizing my troops. Only in this case, my troops were edible. I was an extraordinary strategist. I was the addict in control, not the desperate, emotional, binge-eating freak. I could see my name on the best-seller list with a short description of my book celebrating my exemplary bingeing techniques. And those websites on how to be bulimic had nothing on me.

Bulimia was perfect for my obsessive-compulsive behavior. I thought this addiction was the most wonderful thing that had ever happened to me. I wasn't a drug junkie with needles and sores. I was a food addict with cupcakes and peanut butter chocolate patties..

I used to laugh to myself when I'd think, *I'm feeding my addiction.*

What an appropriate description. How ironic that a heroin junkie was more acceptable to society than a food addict. I could understand, though. Heroin addicts didn't shop in malls or attend high school. And they could be helped, even be cured. Fat girls were out of control, despicable for appearing in public, a curse on the good name of all that was decent in this world – their thin world, of course.

The last part of my bulimic routine culminated in the trip to my bathroom. After bingeing for half an hour, I'd head for the toilet. If I ate more than half an hour, my stomach would rebel. I'd feel actual pain, like it was getting ready to burst. I couldn't go by shape to see if I was full. Too much fat nested in my stomach and abdomen. I looked like I was nine months pregnant all the time.

My body was used to that number of minutes for the first part of my binge-and-purge sessions. Thirty minutes for stuffing the food down, and ten minutes for vomiting was also my lunch time frame. My internal bulimic clock was set.

As I moved like a tidal wave to the bathroom, I congratulated myself on doing everything to perfection. Too bad no one would get to know how talented I was in this area of my life. I could eat as much of anything I wanted, as long as I got it out fast. I was losing weight. Isn't that every girl's dream? I had something to smile about again. I was going to be thin.

Chapter 5

Showtime

In addition to the actual performance of gorging and vomiting, dressing for bulimia at school was vital. I couldn't afford to have vomit splash back on my clothing or shoes. It was trial-and-error at home, until I knew exactly how to protect my clothes at school At home, I could disrobe completely, and then take a shower. I would also wash my hair to make sure nothing had bounced back into it. Even though I was meticulous in how I pushed it back behind my ears before regurgitating, sometimes the spew of food would be explosive. My garbage bag tucked around me in the maintenance shed at school protected me pretty well from that peril. But before I lifted my head away from the toilet bowl at home, I'd make sure the mass in the toilet water hadn't been thrown back into my face and hair before I could flush it. If I was standing instead of kneeling, and I vomited like a fire hose at full pressure, everything in the vicinity would get splattered. When that happened, it would take twice as long to clean as it usually did, because it was all over the walls, the lip of the toilet, the floor and me.

I had to be careful about the noise, too. If the chunks of vomit were pretty big, they would land in the toilet water with an audible splash. It could be rather noisy. It would depend on the height from which the stomach contents were pouring from my mouth. I always turned on the bathroom fan to cover up the puking sounds, but it was worrisome at times when the large solid lumps would drop into the toilet bowl with a huge plop.

I had my clean-up routine well practiced. I had learned from a dreadful experience what can happen if the unexpected, the unplanned, the unanticipated occurred It haunts me still. I was so close to being discovered and losing it all.

The first time I threw up I was worried about the sounds, so I thought I'd empty my stomach completely, and then flush the toilet once. Bad idea. At least diarrhea was liquid, so it would go down like urine. Not so with huge chunks of food. They were like big hard rocks that clogged the toilet drain opening. When I pulled the handle, the mass just sat there for a few seconds, and then it started floating up towards the top of the bowel!

I was in a panic. I hadn't prepared for this. Do I use Mother's towels to catch it? She'd never believe I had gotten that sick from the flu or something I ate.

Hell and damnation! my mind screamed, *what could I do!*

The mounds of food were pushing over the edges of the toilet onto the floor, where I was still kneeling in frozen fear. I looked around for anything I could use as a container. Maybe I could catch the overflow and then flush, so the rest could go down with the biggest hunks out of there. Since I had taken off my glasses, I peered around the bathroom like a senile owl. Everything looked fuzzy. My first thought was about my eyesight:

Now you've done it. You've busted the veins in your eyes. You're going blind, you stupid fat slob. God, you'll be blind and still fat!

Cursing myself helped because I felt bad about myself, anyway, so I could feel free to pour it on when I'd made such a terrible error in my bulimic planning. I could hear Joseph Conrad's degenerate character in **Heart of Darkness** scream, "The horror! The horror!" Of course, my "heart of darkness" wasn't inside me. It was the dark foul mass in the stinking toilet.

Even worse, I thought.

My hands were filled with the goop, as I had tried to catch it and pour it back into the toilet. But since nothing was going down the drain, it just kept coming back up like lava flow. It looked like the volcano in Pompeii that had been so fast it covered people while they were in the act of fleeing. I knew how they felt.

I had drained the water in the tank by desperately pulling on the handle too many times. The handle was flopping up and down, making a tingeing sound against the white top of the toilet tank, to remind me that I would have to wait until the tank had a chance to refill. Although my hands were slick with vomit, I lifted the heavy lid of the tank and grabbed the chain to lift the rubber stopper so the tank would refill more quickly. I just managed to hold onto the heavy lid with one hand, and reach for the chain with the other. Meanwhile, the regurgitated remains of my binge were seeping onto me and dripping onto the bathroom floor with a vengeance. My knees started to slip and slide.

Jesus, what if I lose my balance and hit my head on the toilet bowl. Maybe I'd be knocked out.

Mother would pound on the door.

"You've been in there for over an hour. Is everything alright?"

My father would join her, and start kicking at the door.

"What the hell is going on? Open this damn door!"

The door would crack as his foot and leg fell through. I'd be lying there with my naked, ugly, vomit-covered body sprawled across the bathroom floor. I would look like a gigantic white squid after its final death throes – a fate worse than death. I damn well better be dead if that happened.

Well, it wasn't going to happen if I could help it. I'd find a way out of this. For a moment, I thought I could lap it up and put it back inside me. Anything was better than this stuff carpeting the tile on the bathroom floor. But I realized it would take too long to mop it up in my hands and eat it. It had now covered my hands, and was creeping up my arms. I was scrapping it off with one hand, while holding onto the slimy bowl with the other. Dammit, I needed more hands

I was losing the battle of keeping it off me. Where else could I throw the slabs of regurgitated food? The tub! I began throwing the biggest parts in the tub. Maybe its drain would accommodate more than the one in the toilet. I pulled up the metal stopper, and pushed the vomit down. I turned on the cold water to move the mass along. Some of it was sticking to the sides of the tub and the bottom. I turned on both spigots at the highest pressures. This was becoming a mess of immense proportions, and it was getting ungodly noisy. I could hear it over the bathroom fan. That had never happened before.

I quickly did a once-over of the room to see if there was anything I could use to mask the sound. After washing off my left hand under one of the tub spigots, I pushed one of the large bath towels under the door. The vomit wouldn't reach it if I kept scooping. The shower curtain could be pulled all the way across, to cut down on the noise of the tub spigots running full on and the splashing against the sides of the tub.

I started to panic again. I was running out of things I could do to save myself from the humiliation and shame of having my parents find out what was going on. The water was pouring out from the sink and tub faucets. The tank was filling like it had all the time in the world. I was slipping and sliding in the vomit, trying futilely to keep my knees together so the vomit didn't get caught in the immense fat folds of my thighs. I had turned on the sink faucets without standing. I hoped they didn't overflow. Was the sink stopper up? Too late now to check. Then I happened to look up and see something green on the sink counter.

Yes!

It was a large, lime-green, plastic, drinking cup. Mother always provided oversized objects for me to use, since heavy girls had huge thick hands unable to hold slender items.

I could see the entire cup, if I stood up on my knees just a little bit to give me height from the floor. Fortunately, my vision had cleared a little.

Well, at least I'm not going blind, I thought.

Small comfort at the moment. I made a grab for it. I managed to knock it off. It landed near me and then bounced right next to me. I love plastic!

I used it on the floor like a shovel. It picked up the bathroom contents, and I dumped them in the bathtub. I checked on the level in the toilet tank as I began my assault on the overflowing vomit. I wasn't a perfectionist for nothing. I would get this going strategically.

I scooped with my left hand. I poured the big gobs in the tub and the little ones in the sink. I glanced at the water rising in the tank. I took several of the washcloths that I could rinse out later, unlike the towels, which would have to be washed, and wiped the vomit stuck to the sides of the tub towards the drain.

It was working. I had managed to stop the toilet from overflowing. The largest food blobs had gone down the tub drain. Some of the smaller ones went down the sink drain. The tank was full. I pulled the handle, and the rest of the vomit went its merry way down the toilet drain. With enormous relief, I sat back on my haunches and took several deep breaths. Now I had time to finish cleaning up.

It was imperative there was no sign of what I had done. Heaven forbid, if Mother got the urge to clean my bathroom, and found suspicious stains where none should be.

Okay, I'm in control of this.

First, I made sure the floor was absolutely spotless. I rinsed out the washcloths, and scoured every inch of the tile. I spent at hour scrubbing between the tiles. I checked behind the pipes of the toilet, as well as the obvious areas that were visible. I used an old toothbrush to brush the round sections that were cemented into the concrete of the toilet, sink, and bathtub. Then, when I was satisfied the floor was spotless, I wiped down any counter space and the insides of all the ceramic areas. I made sure to wipe under the lip of the toilet bowl, in addition to the seat knobs where the seat was attached. Anything that might look like barf was scrupulously scrubbed several times. Once the ceramic items were clean, I started on the faucets. I used the toothbrush again around the hard-to-reach areas. I could get the larger metallic portions with the washcloths I kept rinsing and squeezing the water out of. If I could see myself in them, I would know they were free of any coating of food slime. I cleaned the bathroom mirror and replaced the green cup, after I had washed it in hot water numerous times.

Naturally, I didn't use any toilet paper when I upchucked. That was a sure way to clog the toilet. And if I was careless, I might forget and throw it in the basket under the sink, after wiping my food-spattered face, neck, and chest.

So I knew the toilet paper roll was full, but I examined it and the wooden roll like Sherlock Holmes, anyway. You never know. Vomit splatter could hit those, if I had lifted my mouth up a little when I was explosively regurgitating.

Finally, it was time to scrub down the walls. If it was projectile vomit, the food I had consumed last in the binge would come back up in large chunks, and drop like boulders into the toilet water. The stomach acid hadn't had a chance to work on it, so the initial pieces in the vomit could be big and hard. The splash could be monumental, and would thoroughly paint the bathroom walls with gunk. I started at the whiteboards attached to the tile, and made my way up in sections of each wall. The floorboards had indentations in the wood that often caught slivers of vomit that either made brown spots or dripped like a little muddy river down the paint to the bathroom tile. Thanks to my OCD, I felt comfortable checking and re-checking each section of the wall and the wood several times to make sure I hadn't missed a vomit spot.

After washing my bulimic right arm with soap and water up to the elbow, I soaped both hands, and used hot water to rinse. I kept my hands under the water until the skin was bright red. Then I soaped and washed my face with the hottest water I could bear. I grabbed the hand towel hanging on a ring next to me, and scrubbed until my face looked like raw hamburger.

It was like I was punishing myself. Freud would love this.

I had to be careful not to rub too hard on my lips, or the skin would come off. I would have open sores. They were hard to explain, if I hadn't been sneezing around the house so it looked like I had a cold. I could tell Mother the sores were fever blisters from my cold.

I flossed my teeth three times to get any remnants of food caught between them. I brushed my teeth seven times, harder each time, until my gums bled. While putting everything back in its place on the counter, I'd take a big gulp of mouthwash. I'd hold the stinging liquid in my mouth until I had deposited the flossing string in the basket under the sink, and checked the countertop one last time. The mouthwash on my bloody gums hurt like hell. I was an expert at self-abuse. I deserved to suffer. I was ugly and unloved because I was fat. My self-esteem was in the toilet – an apt description, I might add.

No pain, no gain. I chuckled at the perversion of the athlete's code.

After I was convinced the bathroom was pristine, I took a shower for half an hour. I wanted to make sure I found any lingering pieces of regurgitated substances that could hide in my folds of fat. I decided to ask Mother for one of those powerful spray nozzles, so it could cover large surfaces with an impressive amount of power and water pressure. I washed my hair five times. When I had soaped the greatest body areas and used the washcloth to assist the full-on water sluicing down my front and back to get rid of the soap, I lifted up the stomach fat, and looked carefully between my flabby thighs to make absolutely certain nothing was caught in the creases.

My regular-looking upper body had caught up with the obscene lower portions. There was no justice in the world. I couldn't get a break. The hanging flab on my arms would slap against my sides when I scrubbed my front. I would pick up each pendulous breast and run the washcloth under it. My pubic hair was inspected to see if any bits of food had stayed there when I had washed down my front. I ran the washcloth through the crack in my butt several times. I just hoped all the cellulite didn't provide shelter for vomit bits. Craters on the moon couldn't have seemed larger than those on the fronts and backs of my thighs when I was worried about food hiding in them.

When I had finished soaping, washing off, soaping again, and washing off for the third time, I felt ready to step out of the shower for the last part of the cleansing process.

I had already removed the shower mat and toilet seat cover, and stored them under the sink in a small cabinet prior to beginning my purge. Before I had stepped into the shower, I had retrieved them and put them back where they belonged.

I stepped carefully out onto the mat, and stood there toweling myself with several beach towels going at once. It took two to cover my complete body. I used a hand towel to dry my hair.

I had a box of Q-tips in the cabinet behind the mirror above the sink. This was the moment to employ them to the fullest. I did my ears, under my chin, in my bellybutton and between my toes. I had to sit on the edge of the tub to be able to bend over enough to reach my feet. A precarious position, since if I lost my balance and fell back into the tub, I would certainly need help getting out. That couldn't happen. I gripped the shower curtain and leaned forward. I couldn't bring my leg up because of the volume of fat on my calves and ankles; so going over as far as I could was the only way to get to my toes. I did one foot, and then sat back up for an instant. The blood would run to my head when I bent over. I would get really dizzy. When I sat up again, it would take several minutes for my face to return to its usual pale color from the flush of the coagulated blood in my cheeks. Eventually, I would do the other foot. I needed to rest for five to seven minutes before I could stand without keeling over. I kept my grip tightly on the shower curtain at all times.

I wrapped a beach towel around my upper body and tied it. I put another one at my middle to cover my lower areas. Then I walked into my bedroom and just made it to the bed before I collapsed. I was exhausted and breathing through my mouth at this point. I had to lie on my bed for fifteen minutes before I could get up to dress. I also used that time to silently castigate myself.

My God, you idiot. You almost blew it.

I would never make that mistake with the toilet-flushing segment of my bulimic ritual again. Live and learn.

Relief at Last

It was the most gratifying feeling in my bulimic world, when I expunged the food from my binges. The sense of relief was overpowering. I felt wonderful. I had done something great for myself. This was better than anything I had ever experienced before. It was so addictive. And I was really good at this. The best part was that I could do it several times a day, in addition to the school bulimic episodes. I could eat and eat, and still lose weight. I was queen of my own Bulimic Ball.

I had noticed that my fat folds weren't quite as heavy to lift as they usually were, when they would sag over my arms holding them up to search for food particles. I had won the lottery of life. I was ecstatic. I SO wanted to brag to someone, but the fat girls at school wouldn't understand why I'd do that to myself, and the thin girls wouldn't listen to anything I had to say. Mother would have a fit. My father would look at me with revulsion. No, this was something I had to treasure all by myself. No great sacrifice there.

My bulimia at school gave me a thrill. Nobody did it like I did. My bulimic talent was incomparable. The girl-sticks couldn't compete with me in this addictive eating disorder. I had perfected my school bulimic routine to such a fine degree I was in a class by myself. It was such a shame no one could see what I did during the 30 minutes for lunch, that set me apart from everyone else. I was disciplined. I was losing weight at a rapid rate. I would surpass them. My bulimic battle plan at school was superb.

Every day it was the same magnificent bulimic performance. Let me describe the glorious sequence of bulimic events again, just in case I missed a wonderful detail to describe. I can feel the adrenaline rush as I begin. It makes my heart beat faster, and the blood go on a joyride to my face.

When the bell rang to signal the lunch period, I'd head directly for my secret binge-and-purge place. When I arrived and made sure nobody was watching, I snuck into the maintenance shed. It was left open during school hours. The door locked from the outside, so I pushed a chair under the knob just to make sure I was uninterrupted. I got out my bulimia supplies and junk food from my backpack. I laid the food on a white garbage bag I had hidden in a zippered pouch on the side of my backpack. I began my binge. Chocolate, chips, cupcakes, and even some cotton candy I had picked up from a gas station near the school. I crammed them in, then washed them down with the bottle of soda I had purchased along with the junk food.

My taste buds were singing. I closed my eyes to savor the smells. I loved my food. It made me feel warm and wonderful. God, eating was great. I felt a sense of calm and contentment I only got when I was gorging. Normal people didn't know what they were missing. By the time twenty minutes had elapsed, nothing was left to eat. I was full. My stomach ached. It was letting me know the second half of my ritual needed to be started.

I gathered the food wrappings that were all over the plastic I had lain down before I began to binge. I took out another tall, kitchen garbage bag, and deposited the food-package remains in it. I picked up the one on the cement, and tied it around my neck. The tall, kitchen garbage bags were so ideal. I loved those slick red loops that tied together in a plastic bow. The bag worked like an oversized napkin. I kneeled on the cement floor. Kneeling was the most careful way to protect my clothes and shoes. After I had removed my bulimic items from my backpack, I made sure it was placed on the chair holding the door closed. It had to be 'way out of range of any projectile vomit that might miss the plastic covering my lap.

If I had long sleeves in winter, I would roll them over and over up each arm as high as I could, until I felt that I had a makeshift tourniquet on both. I found that if I didn't make them tight enough, the sleeves could slip down at the most inappropriate moment.

When I was bent over in my vomit position, I put my left hand flat on the floor with a stiff elbow to support my weight, and my right hand with a bent elbow naturally curved into a claw. My purge-hand's first two fingers headed for the back of my throat. I was careful not to scrape my knuckles against my front teeth. I had to watch for any sign of a callous there. It was a sure sign of a long-term bulimic.

Usually, it wouldn't take long to start the food back up. My school-regurgitation image I liked the best to get me going was being forced to drink a cup full to the top of excrement, mucus, and large worms. As I peered into the moving contents of the cup, I would visualize the worms' jaws opening as I put the filthy lip of the cup to my mouth. Their sharp teeth were getting ready to slice through my lip as my head was pushed into the cup. The fat worms moved around in the muck like the Lock Ness monster. There was no way to avoid them getting hold of me. No area of the cup was worm-free. The thick rings around their necks let me know where their heads were. Yellow cataracts covered their eyes. The worms would suck up some of the snot, and then look up at me. It didn't take long for my lunch binge to start to come back up when I got going with this graphic mental aid.

The worm-cup was my primary visualization. But if my stomach was particularly full, I'd use the one that was even quicker to work to get purging. I would be strapped to a table. It was made from unfinished wood. Large splinters pushed themselves into my body whenever I tried to move. My head would be held in place by heavy steel clamps that bit into my scalp. My jaw was abnormally stretched with an old leather belt pulling down on it. The ends of the belt were nailed into the wood table on each side. Pincer-like tongs were attached to my eyelids. They were so heavy they could be laid down on my forehead and do their job. I couldn't close my eyes or my mouth. Above my head was a big bowl attached to a pulley. In the bowl lay a bloody birth placenta with a long umbilical-looking stalk, coated with thick red and yellow gobs of slime-like pus. When I looked up, the bowl would be tipping towards my face. The heavy blood-engorged placenta was sloshing to the edge. Its thick stalk hung over. The layered liquid coating it began to ooze downward. In a second, it would drip into my stretched, wide-open mouth.

Usually I'd be vomiting into the garbage bag before the placenta landed in my mouth. Unlike the jaw worms, I didn't have to create the unappetizing afterbirth picture

We had seen one in a film in Biology. Everyone in the room had gagged.

Great Little Secrets

Mother noticed my weight loss one day when we were passing on the stairs. She automatically moved against the wall. But this time I got by her without too much trouble.

"I see your diet is working. I have a little secret to share with you. I asked my friends at work how they stay so slim. Several of them told me about the diet doctors who help them with medication. Each Saturday they go for their weekly shot. I thought we'd see if it would help you lose weight a little faster."

The next Saturday we arrived early at a building that seemed to be an odd place for a clinic.

"Mother, are you sure this is the place? I don't see any medical stuff on the building."

Mother peered at the address in her hand.

"Janice said it was a little hard to find. Let's look around back"

As we rounded the corner, we ran into a long line of girls waiting next to a series of folding tables. They looked like tables in a bingo hall. There were women sitting behind them in everyday clothes. In front of them were separate piles of hypodermics and alcohol pads. Nothing else. No blood-pressure cuffs or stethoscopes. I couldn't see anyone who looked like a doctor. No white smocks with laminated name badges anywhere. Well, it was a Saturday. The women seemed professional as they maneuvered the medical supplies in front of them.

Mother approached the last girl in line who was standing next to her mother. I liked this girl right away. She was fatter than I was.

"Is this the clinic that gives the shots?"

"Yeah, this is it. You have to fill out that pink sheet before they'll give it to you, though."

Mother picked up one from the large stack on the last table in the row. There wasn't anyone to ask about the form. Mother and I read it over. It was the standard form that asked if you had any health problems.

"Well, you're in good health. Check all the boxes 'no.' I'll sign at the bottom for you."

"Mother, it says in small print here that there are some serious side effects, and they won't take any liability if you sign it."

Mother was getting a little annoyed with me.

"Don't worry. I'm sure they have to list everything that could happen and never does."

I shut up and got behind the girl fatter than I was. I definitely liked that a lot. Her mother and mine began to talk about the shots. I listened as the line began to move forward.

"Jessica used to weigh over 300. She's down to 280 after coming here for the last month."

I liked the sound of that. She lost 20 pounds in one month! I'd lose weight even faster, since I was bulimic, too. This was great. Mother had finally found a way to show she cared about me.

And that's how I added another addiction to the one I had.

We shuffled forward like bovines moving through the chute to the end where a bar drops down to hold their heads in place while they get inoculated. I felt like bellowing "Moo," but Mother was already ticked at me. I didn't think she would find my comment amusing.

The lady at the first table took the pink form from Mother, and put it in a bunch next to her without reading it. So much for their concern about any health conditions you might have checked on their no-liability paper.

As we were headed for the next tables with the syringes, I noticed the fat girls in front of me were pulling down their pants so their hips were exposed on the side nearest the tables. Jessica jerked hers down quickly. It would have been funny if I had paused to consider what we looked like, with our fat hips displayed like slabs of processed meat waiting for the butcher to stamp Grade A.

The line was going pretty fast now. I watched as each girl waited for the alcohol pad, and then the hypo. If you wanted one, band-aids in various sizes were scattered among the empty needles. Most girls wanted to get their pants back up as soon as the needle came out. They hadn't worn any underwear that I could see. Many showed small spots of blood on the outside of their clothing where they'd gotten the shot. There was no stopping the factory-like line. Sometimes, the girls still hadn't gotten their pants up over their hips before they arrived at what I called the Checkout table. Without looking up, a lady put out her hand, and the mothers put twenty dollars in it. Mother had heard it was a "cash only" setup. Should have been a clue right there that this was an illegal operation.

The woman with her hand out for the money said the same exact words to everyone when they handed off the drug payoff. That was funny when I thought about it. We were middle-class, social drug junkies.

She still didn't look up as she printed out the receipt, and said in a monotone:

"Wait here for ten minutes to make sure you don't have any bad reactions."

What would they do if we did? There weren't any doctors around. I didn't think the table ladies were nurses. There wasn't even a table with little white paper cups of orange juice, like you get when you give blood. Of course there wouldn't be any cookies on it anyway, considering the reason we all were there.

No one waited around. It was probably the liability thing again for her to tell us to wait ten minutes. I guess if you had a seizure at the eleventh minute, they took no responsibility.

It was my turn in line. I pulled down my pants to expose my hip. I thrust it towards the table next to me. The shot was over in a minute. She never looked up at my face. I didn't even look at the place where she had injected me. I didn't care if I was bleeding. Everything I wore now was black (the "slimming" color, according to Mother), so the blood wouldn't show anyway. Besides, putting a band-aid on meant I had to leave my flesh exposed for a longer period of time. No way that was going to happen.

Mother whispered to me as I pulled up my jeans:

"Here's the money." She put two tens in my hand.

Soon I was through with the whole process. I wondered what was in the shot.

"Mother, what do the hypos have in them?"

Mother looked nervously at the others behind us.

"It's some powerful drug that will help with your appetite."

Okay. I knew about amphetamines. Now I had just been injected with one.

My heart began to race as I climbed in the car and buckled up for the ride home.

Mother glanced sideways at me.

"Do you feel any different?"

Yeah, like I was at the starting gate of the Kentucky Derby, juiced up and ready to gallop. I liked this feeling. In fact, I LOVED this feeling.

"Yes, I feel like I'm on an energy high."

Mother looked blank for a minute.

"Is that what it is supposed to do?"

I don't think Mother had ever heard of amphetamines, even though she'd been addicted to them for years. Her doctors called them stimulants. Like drinking several cups of coffee in a row, she told me once. Just to get her going in the morning. She had noticed some brown pills I had accidentally left on the kitchen counter one day.

"Those are pretty big vitamins."

"Yeah, they're helping me with my diet. I got them in the health food section at the store."

As soon as she heard the word "diet," Mother lost interest. I was always on a diet. That was a good thing. My parents thought it was normal for fat girls to be forever on diets to improve their appearance.

Actually, the oblong brown pills were 500 milligrams of caffeine tablets, the only jump-start a minor could get. I'd throw down a couple before I went to school. I bought the largest bottles they had. Fortunately, in case Mother caught a glimpse of one, they looked like the organic vitamin containers Mother had at home. They made me a bit edgy, but I could keep refining my bulimia at a more rapid pace when I took them.

Now I had found the ultimate drug high to go along with my other addiction. Well, Mother had found it for me. This was terrific. I had the energy to eat and vomit continually without worrying about sleep. I didn't trust the drug to do everything for me. I needed my bulimia. I was sure about that. No sense taking chances. What if the shot didn't last all week? I could still lose weight with my tried-and-true method. I still wanted my junk food. I probably wouldn't binge as often. That was okay since it was such a pain to make sure I wasn't caught, and I didn't enjoy the clean-up part as much as the bingeing and purging portions of my bulimic sessions. The injections were cleaner and quicker. I decided this weekly shot was going to be a great companion for my first love – bulimia. Now I had two best friends.

Toasting My Success

With my amphetamine injections, I stayed thin for my first two years of college while I lived with my parents. Mother paid for the shots. But in my junior year, I decided I could handle living in a dorm. I had a second-hand car Mother had found for me from one of the neighbors. A lady who lived down the street from us was selling her son's old car, since he was headed off to an out-of-state college. I could commute to the diet clinic myself from the campus.

Just to be sure I stayed rail-thin at school, I ate one meal a day at a restaurant that saved the heels of loaves of bread for me. That's what I ate for two years – four pieces of toast and diet sodas. God, I was so thin. I loved it. Sometimes I'd get tired during the day, but when the girls gave me appraising glances and the guys wanted to talk to me, the last thing on my mind was dropping dead from malnutrition. I never believed the propaganda about how any body-type was fine. That's beyond ludicrous. I knew how people really felt.

I could remember that when I started to gain weight, my father had told me my butt looked like two cats fighting in a bag. It was an off-hand remark. Of course it became the reason I became a food addict. I was ugly, even to my father. He seldom paid the attention Mother did to my looks. I knew how things were, right then and there. If I wasn't perfect, he wouldn't love me. My OCD brain kicked into action on the weight front. It was all downhill from there.

The truth is the real world doesn't like fat people. It treats them like the leftovers you throw out when they begin to rot. When a girl is fat, she is not the main dish. You got it. She's the leftover. My father just said what the world already thought. No big deal. Unless your mother is mentally ill, and you inherited her disease. Bring on the addictive behavior. I only needed to finally understand how I could be loved. Good ol' dad put it into words. I had to be thin to earn affection. I would be so thin so he would have to love me.

I was still in honor classes at the university, but I didn't have to depend on the people in them to have friends, especially boyfriends. When you're slender, the whole world bows down. Lots of guys wanted to get into my lacy bikini panties. I could get into a car wreck, and my mother would be proud of me for what the EMTs would see underneath my clothes. Those EMTs would want to keep me all for themselves, and would flirt outrageously on the way to the hospital.

I created my own little fantasy about it. Even though I was only slightly injured, my clothes would have to be removed. It was orgasmic just thinking about the television-handsome ER doctor carefully cutting down the front of my top to my skinny little bottom. He would want to make passionate love to me right there behind the curtains. I knew this was how it would happen.

The Real Thing

In the school library, I had spent most of my adolescent life reading countless romantic novels with plots like the one I had seen myself in. But I discovered I had something better at home than those bland predictable tales. Our house had an attic with an old mattress and a door that locked. Hours were spent with flushed-face salivating over the pages of my father's soft porn I had found in his underwear drawer. I made sure I was always around when Mother washed his underwear, so

I could put it away in his chest of drawers. That way, I could access his new stash of sex novels without suspicion.

I brought an old bed coverlet from my bedroom to put over the mattress. I'd lie there for hours, reading page after page of paperbacks with titles like, "Hot Nurses on Call" or "Hot Love in a Hot Tub." The titles were indicative of the writing expertise, too. It wasn't Tolstoy. But it was the sex scenes I focused on. These authors knew what their audiences wanted. The plots just led to one sex act after another.

I only took one book at a time from my father's underwear drawer. I always put it back before he got home. And I made sure it was in the exact spot it was in before I borrowed it. My perfectionism paid off here, too. My father never caught on. 'Though my mother probably saw them, she would never mention them to my father. She probably thought all married men had them. Their little "men" secret.

Since I was brainy, it didn't take long for my body to catch up after reading a particularly salacious sex act over and over. I'd bunch up the blanket, shove it between my legs, and let my imagination do the rest. Pretty soon, I was rising and falling off that mattress, as if electric shocks were being administered. Arching and moaning, I'd smother my face in the mattress so the sounds didn't penetrate the attic door.

As careful as I was, sometimes my libido would take complete control. I'd be writhing all over the mattress, arching my back, digging my heels into the soft form and screaming for all I was worth.

"What's going on up there?"

Mother had passed by the door and heard the sounds of my "blanket orgasms."

Gasping for air, it would take me a minute to answer her.

"Nothing, Mother. I was moving some boxes around and stubbed my toe."

"Well, be careful."

I would wait breathlessly for her to move on.

My God, what wonderful times those were! But now I was in college, I wanted the real thing. It was all around me. Guys with their shirts off playing basketball; runners with small silky shorts racing past me with their genitals moving behind those jockstraps. Men coming out of the other girls' dorm rooms in the early morning, their zippered crotches gazing hard at me as we passed in the hallway.

Chapter 6

My Turn

It was definitely time to get some. And I had choices, now that I was one of the thins. An orgy would have been okay by me, but I finally narrowed it down to two. One was in one of my classes. The other was screwing a blonde down the hall from my room. Since it might be a little much for me to grab the one screwing near me in the dorm room two doors from mine, I decided I'd shoot for the one in one of my classes. If he wasn't interested, it wouldn't be such a big deal, since this was the last scheduled class for this course. I wouldn't see him again, anyway.

I had lusted over him all semester. He sat in front of me, so I could look at him leisurely. His wide shoulders, hairy legs in cargo shorts, and the hair curling on the back of his neck, were tantalizing. I wanted to jump him right there and then. It was so hard to concentrate on the subject, especially since my eyes were more attracted to his butt than my book. It was an elective course, anyway, to fulfill the science requirement. Someone had told me Geology was the easiest one to take.

Instead of paying attention to the lectures on rocks, I started fantasizing what it would be like to have him rock-hard inside me. It would be like the graphic sex in my father's porn novels. I knew I had to have him, or I was going to fail my class. Already my body was causing problems. I knew my pupils were enlarged, my clitoris was engorged, and I was leaking into my panties. It didn't help that my jeans were so tight that if I crossed my legs, the zipper would be crushed against my labia. If I moved at all, I was heading for a giant orgasm right there in class. It was all I could do to think of my dog dying to get me to calm down.

The professor glanced around the room.

"Does anyone have any questions?"

No one had any questions. I don't think a question was asked all semester. If I hadn't had the stud in front of me to fantasize about, I'd have had a terrible time staying awake. Geology might be the easiest course to pass, but it was also the most boring.

"Remember that the rock cleavages are different, depending on the composition of the rock."

This last lecture was not helping.

I'd love to have that rock-hard chest pressed to my cleavage. I'd run my fingers along his spine until I reached his...

I had to do something fast. I pushed my book off my desk. Picking it up would let me unlock my legs, and get the damn zipper away from my most vulnerable body area.

He turned and looked down at the book near my desk.

He looked from it to me and smiled when he picked it up and handed it to me.

"Yeah, I feel the same way," he said in a low voice as the professor wound down his lecture.

It was now or never.

"Would you like to have a cup of coffee, to compare notes for the final? I don't think I was listening half the time today," I said.

Thinking about you moving in me kept me totally occupied, I thought.

My mouth curved into a smile I hoped wasn't too lascivious.

"Sure. Let's go over to the Student Union."

Yes!

"Great. Thanks for the help. Is this your major?"

I made small talk as we walked together across the quad. I didn't hear a thing he said. His body so close to mine was taking me to whole new places in my brain.

While we chatted, I was really concentrating on the great thigh muscles in those washed out jeans he was wearing SO well.

I listened with half an ear, as he talked about the prospects for the basketball team. I was hoping that wasn't all he was thinking about. My knee had bumped his several times while we were talking.

"Maybe we could get together later. I share an apartment with a couple of guys not far from the campus."

I should play it coyly. Hell with that. I wanted to get laid.

"Sounds like a plan."

"I'll pick you up at your dorm, and we can walk over. Would 8:30 tonight be okay?"

Oh yeah.

"Yes, that would be fine."

All right!

He would come in and sign for me. Heaven would open its pearly gates. I was one of the thins who had hot guys meet them in the dorm foyer. I just about wet my pants with excitement.

Or was it something else making me wet.

Nasty girl.

It was really going to happen, and all because I was thin like other college coeds, who had probably had sex since they were in high school. The football jocks and the cheerleaders – it was such a cliché. But I was so envious of those smirks on their faces, when they got to school late the next day after a football game. I could almost smell the sex on them.

Now, it was my turn to become a woman, by having some guy I barely knew plow through my thickened hymen like a barracuda in heat. I couldn't wait. I wanted that next-morning "I had sex" smile. I had earned it with my toast-and-soda diet, that left my stomach pressed close to my spine. I could almost reach around my waist with both hands. Scarlett O'Hara had nothing on me, and I wasn't even tied into a corset to get that 18-inch waist. I wanted to look sophisticated and smug because I, too, knew the secret of sex. It was tough waiting for the clock hands to get to 8:30.

I think his name was Brad or Greg. It didn't really matter. As long as he had the requisite equipment for the job, he was in (in more ways than one, I hoped).

Everything went SO slowly until the time I would see whatever-his-name was.

Having sex with myself in the attic with a rolled-up blanket was going to be enthusiastically replaced by the real thing. I could hardly keep my skinny thighs from spasmodically clenching with anticipation.

I almost ejaculated right there in the dorm foyer, when I saw him after they buzzed me I had a visitor. He was wearing a V-necked, black t-shirt and a newer pair of washed out jeans. He had on Vans with no socks. Some of his chest hair showed, where the collar allowed. It was a shirt easy to get off fast. Now I understood the phrase, "He looked good enough to eat."

Yeah, boy!

Walking to his apartment took about twenty minutes.

"My roommates are at the gym for a couple of hours."

Terrific!

And, I might add, he looked like he worked out, too. His biceps pushed the shirt material towards the top of his arms. Bet that stomach was a six-pack. I imagined every part of him was well muscled. I was getting worked up just thinking about what lay beneath those clothes. My breasts started to swell, and my nipples stabbed my bra. Damn. All those romance passages had it right so far – bulging anything on him led to wet swollen parts on mine.

"Would you like something to drink?"

"Water would be great, thanks."

I watched as he walked into the small kitchen and opened the refrigerator. *God, he moved well. Great butt, too.*

"So how do you like Geology?"

I smiled, keeping my eyes focused on the big hand closed around the glass of water he was bringing me.

Big hands, big feet, big….

"The best part of that class is, it's over."

Actually, the BEST part was you. Was it getting hot in here?

I think my eyes gave me away. As he handed me my glass of water, my eyes were at crotch level on him. I couldn't glance away. He leaned over to kiss me, and I pulled him down on the couch. I opened my mouth, so our tongues touched. He got the message my body was sending.

Ten minutes later our clothes were on the floor around his bed.

I let him go long enough for him to reach into his side table drawer for a condom.

I watched impatiently as he put it on his enormous cock. I knew that big bulge in the front of his jeans was for real.

He moved between my legs. I drew my knees up.

"Wow, you're really wet."

He had the most glorious penis. Long and hard. Its circumcised head knew just where to go. I opened my legs as wide as I could. He took one hand and guided it in.

Yes!

"Jesus, you're so tight."

He grunted with pleasure as he thrust, came back out, and was poised to come back in. I couldn't wait.

My legs and butt seemed to have minds of their own. I grabbed his waist and lifted my hips, so he could come in fast. I felt this pain and counted to five. It went away. He was through. I was officially a woman!

It was like a page from a soft-porn romance tableau. I got his rhythm and moved with him as he pounded away.

"I'm coming!"

I felt his pulsating penis empty itself, as the muscles in my vagina squeezed him dry.

He collapsed on top of me, breathing hard. I loved the dampness between my legs. He lifted himself, looked down past his wet pubic hair, and removed the full condom. He showed it to me before he took it to the bathroom. I had a last look at his gorgeous ass, before I thought to look down at myself. I sat up and peered between my thighs. I didn't see anything that looked like bloody tissue. My mind started racing.

God, I hope I haven't bled all over his sheets.

I frantically scanned the sheets.

Nothing but a wet spot.

I had noticed there was nothing of me left on his cock when he removed the condom.

Where the hell is the hymen? Should I look for it? Maybe it's shoved up in there.

I didn't want to take the chance it could pop out like a slick fish onto his bed. I rolled off to the side, careful to keep my legs together.

I couldn't believe this was happening. Why wasn't this explained in those porn books? I should have asked my roommate.

But then she would know I hadn't had sex. Couldn't do that. She talked about her sex life constantly.

I grabbed my panties and bra and quickly put them on. At least if it decided to show itself, I had some layers between it and the rest of the world. If I could get back to the dorm without showing anything, I'd start going to church.

I shouted at the closed bathroom door:

"Hey, I've got to go."

Now what do I say? A thank-you seemed appropriate, but I wasn't sure that was the thing to say after being reamed for an hour.

I looked at the closed door for an instant.

Oh, what the hell. I WAS thankful.

"Thanks!" I bolted out of there, and almost ran back to the dorm. I was afraid to look down, as I made it to the foyer, into the elevator, and up to my room.

I locked myself in our bathroom, and sat on the toilet. I felt something start to slide towards the bowl. It was the torn hymen. I flushed it.

See, I was right. God loves skinny girls. I was saved from certain embarrassment. A semester of countless sex acts was awaiting me. Practice makes perfect. And I was known for doing things perfectly. Thank God for bulimia and uppers. They got me skinny, so I could have real sex. Who could ask for more?

On the weekends, I'd visit the local drinking hangouts around the campus. You knew you were at a university from the amount of bars and tattoo parlors.

I had a ritual I used that got me lots of sex. First, I'd go in the bar within walking distance of my dorm. I didn't have any trouble getting in, since my low-cut blouse and slender legs in my tight denim skirt made me immediately eligible for admittance to the smoke-filled, music-blaring bar. After I entered, undulating my hips as I model-stepped in front of the bouncer, I would lean on the doorjamb next to him for a moment while I scoped out the room.

Sometimes the bouncers would ask me to wait until the bar closed, and then we'd go back to their apartments. The bouncers were muscular, and I really liked thinking about how those muscles were best put to work for me, but I often didn't want to wait for my sex fix.

If I saw a good candidate at the bar for my sex binge, I'd make my way towards him. The tables weren't as dependable for hooking the guy. He'd either be waiting for his girl to come back from the bathroom if he was sitting alone, or he'd be sitting with a bunch of guys, and it would be more work to separate him from the pack.

The bar was the fastest way to get what I needed. I'd perch on the stool next to the stud I wanted, and order. If I caught his eye when I was ordering, he'd buy the next round. Each time I drank a little, I'd lean over more and more, until he was looking at my chest. As I crossed my legs, my skirt would pull up to mid- thigh. I'd hold my drink in one hand, take an ice cube out with the other, and suck on it while I talked with him. I had seen that move on television and in the movies lots of times. It always worked for the girls in the advertisements or up on the screen. I guess the guy fantasized about her sucking something else, with as much energy and finesse as she was going at that ice cube.

When I thought it was time to get him out of there with me, I'd put my empty glass down, and my hands would go to his bicep and thigh. His pupils would contract, and he knew he had a hot invitation.

"It's getting a little hot in here, don't you think?" I'd ask, as my hand slid up and down the inside of his leg.

"Maybe we could go somewhere…" I didn't have to say anything else.

He'd holler for the bartender to pay our tabs. While he was getting the bills out of his wallet, I'd brush my breast against his forearm as he extended it to pay.

As we left the bar, I'd put his arm around my waist. If his hand went lower, I could feel the heat coming to a boil between my legs. I couldn't get him to his place fast enough. Usually, he'd break the speed limit, as my hand would run from his knee up towards his groin, and his foot on the accelerator would involuntarily press down.

When we got to his off-campus apartment, we were silent as we walked through the door. Like the first time, I sat on the couch while he made some drinks for us. I wasn't really interested in his bar, just his body. When he gave me my glass, I touched his fingers and rubbed them across the knuckles. He took my drink, and set both of them down on his coffee table. He pulled me up, and crushed me to him. I gave him a deep, tongue-lashing kiss while his hands began to unbutton my blouse. I reached for his jeans' zipper. We discarded clothes while we moved into his bedroom. I could have written this script for a Hollywood movie when I pushed him down on the bed, and moved my knee gently into his groin. He moaned, and one hand reached for a side drawer in the lamp table next to his king-sized bed. By this time we were naked, and the warmth from our bodies could have lit up the room better than his electric lights ever could. I could feel my nipples swelling and tender to his touch. As he mouthed them, I reached for his engorged penis. My fingers traced the big vein from the top down to the head and up again. He rolled over, and put on the condom. I was waiting with knees spread wide open for his return. He and I rose up to meet. I had been wet from the moment I had fondled his thigh in the bar, so it wasn't long until we had the bed making noises to equal our own as we moved all over it.

When we were finished, I felt wonderful. I was still tingling from his body. He removed the condom and went into the bathroom. I lazily watched his buttocks contract as he walked across the carpet.

After flushing the condom, he came back and put himself next to me on top of the sheet. He fell asleep with his head on my chest. I was tempted to stay there with him. He felt so good. But I had to get back to the dorm by midnight. So I slid out from under him, got dressed as quietly as I could, gave him a kiss on the nape of his neck, called a cab with my cell phone in his living room, and then went outside to wait for it, so I could get back to my dorm on time.

This became my routine for several months. Often, I wouldn't bother asking their names, since I wouldn't be seeing them again, anyway. I liked the hunt, so I didn't want to settle for a boyfriend, when I could have many different experiences with all kinds of healthy males.

I learned how to use my own body, so I could get multiple orgasms with my many partners, if they weren't skilled enough or couldn't wait long enough for me to get off. I knew this was another addiction. I didn't care. I looked attractive, and entered the world of "hooking up" as quickly as was possible.

If the weather was warm enough, and it usually stayed hot till November, I'd throw a blanket in my car so I could take my lovers out in the desert. I'd suggest that we take my car since I knew a great spot to watch the stars. He'd get a bottle for us from the bar, and we'd be on our way. While I was driving, I'd move my legs apart so my short skirt would slide provocatively up towards my slit. If I was especially sex-starved, I would have removed my panties while he was getting our portable liquor.

While we were racing down the desert highway, I'd take looks at him to see when he'd start glancing at my legs. When I knew his eyes were focused on my short skirt, I'd quickly get the denim material on its rapid journey up my thighs until it hit the treasure trove. Even in the dark, I could feel the heat from his body as he slid over the leather seats and placed his hand on my exposed thigh. If I moved just right, I could get his fingers just where I wanted them. He'd put his other hand inside my blouse. Of course, I never wore bras on my sex trips. He'd be working both ends at the same time.

My driving would become a bit erratic at that point. As he squeezed my breasts and fingered my clitoris, I was occupied with one hand on the steering wheel and the other on his crotch. I'd run my fingers up his engorged penis under his jeans. Then I'd go for his belt and zipper. I discovered I was really dexterous with that one hand. It usually took me less than a minute to get his zipper down and have my hand inside his jeans outside his underwear. His mouth was all over my neck and ear, and his fingers had moved from my swollen labia to inside me. As I put my hand around his huge penis and pulled it out through the front hole in his underwear, he'd be thrusting his two fingers then three fingers in and out of my wet-lipped labia.

As I squeezed and ran my fingers over the big vein in his penis, I'd encircle the head and catch the pre-cum. I'd lift my saturated fingers and put them in my mouth and suck. By this time, he was panting and groaning. Since I needed him inside me, I didn't want to take the chance he'd ejaculate before I got what I wanted. I knew where the old dirt roads were, so I put on my brights and looked for the next one.

I wasn't long until one showed up ahead. I pulled the car off the highway and headed down the dust-covered road. When we'd hit a bump, I'd let out a scream. His fingers would go further inside while his thumb rubbed my clitoris. I would have my hand back on his penis and when the car jumped, I'd spasmodically grip it. When I couldn't wait another second, I stopped the car, grabbed the blanket from the back seat, and pulled him from the car.

If I couldn't wait to find a rock slab or place to lie down away from the cactus and little rocks, I'd spread the blanket on the ground next to the car and drop down on it with him.

It took less than a minute for us to be out of our clothes, especially me, since I wasn't wearing any underwear. Men are usually fast to get out of their jeans, especially when their belts and zippers are already taken care of, and their shirts come off over their heads in an instant.

His hands were all over me. Mine were doing the same with him. I roughly rolled him on his back and mounted him. God, he felt wonderful! His hands moved to my breasts and kneaded them. The one hand went between my legs and gently squeezed my clitoris as my finders raked his balls. Every time I went up, I slammed down on his rock-hard pulsing penis. I rode him for all he was worth.

I could feel him getting ready to explode inside me as the walls of my vagina squeezed his gigantic organ.

"Wait, wait! Just a minute more, baby!"

He was groaning as I moved my hips from side to side to have that great piece of meat rub against my walls. I raised myself one last time so his penis was just touching my outer swollen labia. He tried to pull me back on him. I looked down and reveled in the sight of his abnormally large penis moving back and forth across my pubic hair while it searched for my opening. It was slick with my fluids and pulsated as its tip found the opening.

"Please, please!" He was begging.

I couldn't wait another second, but I made it slow, so I could savor every inch of him. He was pushing up his hips and his hands were on my ass pulling me down. I grabbed them and put them on my hard nipples. I lowered my chest to his mouth, still keeping him from fully filling me. As he palmed my nipples and then pulled them towards his mouth, I let him in a little more. The more he sucked, the more he was allowed to be pulled in by my wet squeezing vagina. As he bit one nipple and then the other, I couldn't stand it anymore and came down all the way to his hot balls.

"Oh baby, oh my God…" He yelled.

I felt the orgasm building and it reached its peak as he hit the back of my uterus and exploded inside. His massive load of semen gushed and filled me as I pumped him. My orgasm hit at the same time and our fluids mixed and dripped out and onto his pubic hair and stomach. I held him inside until I got every last drop from that wonderful organ. We were both panting like we had just finished a marathon.

A sex marathon. ·I liked that.

After we did it on the hood of my car doggie style, I let him put his clothes back on, redressed myself, had a drink from the bottle he'd bought, and then drove him back to the bar. I'd give him a long kiss and then accelerate out of the parking lot. These particular desert sex romps were repeated as often as I could fit them in around my schooling. Just thinking about them got me through some long class sessions at the university.

I had always loved the desert. In a funny way, it was loving me back with all the men I had under that gorgeous night sky on that expansive desert floor. I was having a hellava good time, and since I wasn't wasting a lot of time eating meals while I was out hunting for sex, my calorie intake stayed low. Besides, I was getting protein from the semen I swallowed during my 69 trysts.

For the very first time, I loved my life. I was happy, satiated, and open for any adventure my men could come up with. Often, I was the one with the creative positions and techniques. The **Kama Sutra** had nothing on me. I could have added a chapter or two.

It was a good thing I made it a point to have as many lovers as I could. I was about to return to a place I thought I'd never be again. I should have known. It was too good to last.

Crash and Burn

The diet clinic closed down. They weren't there one day when I arrived for my weekly shot. Mother learned later it was not a legitimate medical clinic. But by that time, I was hooked. I thought my world was coming to an end. I had lost half my body weight. Though I was jittery and hyper from the shot, I could cut down on my messy and time-consuming bulimic episodes. And it was getting harder to disguise them in the dorm.

If I wanted, when I was alone and felt like it, and I wasn't gorging on my lovers, I could chow down on pizza and hamburgers any time of the day or night, and throw it all back up in the restaurants' restrooms. The whole process of eating and regurgitating would take at the most 30 minutes. I wasn't even late for "lights out," or any of my classes. And the amphetamines slashed my appetite, and let me do "all nighters" for tests and papers. I had the best of all possible diet worlds.

Now what was I going to do? I had to have my weekly fix. I knew the old story. I'd gain back the weight I'd lost and more. I didn't think bulimia alone could save me. I'd have to vomit twenty times a day. That was an impossibility at school. And I noticed some of my sex dates were looking at me a bit suspiciously when I'd excuse myself to go to the bathroom after eating with them if they were hungry, if we did that before going to their places or the desert for sex.

Oh my God! I wouldn't have any boyfriends again.

Fat girls study in the library all night; they don't get invited to parties and boys' apartments or have heavy sex parties in the desert.

My world was crashing. I felt trapped. Maybe Mother could help. She was an expert at finding doctors who would give her what she wanted. She was a drug addict before it had a name. Instead of treating her for clinical depression and anxiety, the doctors dosed her with pills. She was already an alcoholic, before she brought other drugs into the mix. No wonder her moods were so severe. Most people would be dead from what she took each day. She didn't know any other way to get through the day. I could relate, although I had tried vodka and didn't like the taste.

I didn't communicate with her often. If I called, she'd get going about her countless injustices. When I stopped by, it was to get something from my room that I could use in the dorm. I visited during the day when everyone was out. They hadn't seen me for months. But this was an emergency. I called when I knew she would be home from work.

"Mother, do any of your friends get some chemical help so they can stay thin?"

I had to be more specific. She wasn't answering me on the phone. She was getting more and more forgetful. It was probably the addictions. If you used alcohol and drugs at the levels she did, it was bound to take its toll on your brain cells as well as your liver.

"Like the shots, Mom."

It finally clicked. She knew what I wanted.

"You know, Betty, the new girl in the office told us about a new diet drug that just came out. She says it's wonderful. She even forgets to eat because she says she has no appetite."

This sounded too good to be true.

"Do you remember where she got it?"

I could hear her putting the phone down.

"Mother, are you still there?"

Had she zonked out while I was talking with her? It had happened before, at home. She'd be speaking to someone and in the middle of the conversation, she'd drop the phone and walk off. My father got an answering machine, and would try to get to the telephone before she could if it rang while he was at home. I would do the same, if I was visiting them. Just another day with Mother.

"I'm here. I had to go get the address from my purse."

"Mother, did you get a doctor's name or telephone number?"

A long pause. I began to get worried.

"Yeah, it's at the bottom of the card Betty gave me."

She read off the number. The line went dead.

I redialed as fast as I could. It rang several times, and then she picked up. I hadn't realized I was gripping the phone like it was the last one on planet Earth, until I happened to look down at my hand. It looked bloodless from how hard my fingers were wrapped around the receiver.

"Hello?" Her voice sounded far away.

"Mother, are you all right?"

"Of course. I'm fine. Why are you asking me that?"

I had to be careful here. If she heard what she thought was an accusatory tone, she'd get defensive and start in with me about how dad and I didn't trust her, or think she couldn't do anything. She had obviously forgotten I had just spoken with her.

"I was just checking to see if you needed anything. I could stop by after my last class."

"No. We don't need anything."

"Okay, I'll talk to you later." I was speaking to dead air. She had already hung up.

Well, at least I knew she was still functioning.

I called the number Mother had given me, and made an appointment for the next day. I just hoped the effects of my last weekly shot would hang in there until I could get another option. I vomited every time I put food in my mouth. Even tic-tacs came back up. I wasn't taking any chances.

The next morning, I went to my classes and then drove across town to the address the receptionist had given me. She had also told me to bring $60.00 in cash. No checks or credit cards. This sounded familiar and promising.

When I walked in, I breathed a sigh of relief. I recognized a diet den when I saw one. There were so many anorectic-looking girls in the waiting room they could have all fitted on one couch. One had her leg turned so far behind her other one, it seemed I was seeing just one. Balanchine would have loved this room, whether these girls danced or not. Bony protuberances were everywhere. Bones rubbing against bones. I was in the right place. There was a sign on the reception desk: "Payment Must Be Made at Time of Service." Underneath, the amount was listed for the visit - $60 cash. No credit cards or checks accepted.

I grinned when I saw the form on the circular desk. It was the same as the one I filled out at the diet clinic. I was home.

It was like a diet-office conveyer belt. I thought of those moving sidewalks at theme parks.

The receptionist/guide would say:

"Now, here on your left is your pink health form. I mean our 'get-rid-of-fat' card."

She would giggle and put her anorectic hand over her mouth after collecting the entrance fee.

"When you see an open door, please step off and go through it. Your diet doctor will be waiting."

As I sat down in one of the waiting room chairs, I chuckled to myself as I envisioned these skin-and-bone girls looking for their doors on the moving diet clinic walkway.

I would discover that I wasn't far off the mark with my fantasy scenario. As I signed my pink form, the bony hand of the clinic's receptionist reached for it, took it in her skinny fingers, and dropped into a metal basket on her desk. It wasn't a good idea to have overweight receptionists in diet clinics. It didn't bode well for the product.

As I walked away, I noticed that she didn't read it to see if I had checked any of the diseases listed on one side. The only thing she glanced at on the form was the signature beneath the "No liability" clause. Hmm, seemed familiar. Another action that showed I was in the right place.

Every ten minutes, a girl's name was called. She'd disappear down a hallway, open one of the seven doctors' doors, go in, and come back out about fifteen minutes later with a prescription in her hand.

I could tell my amphetamine shot had worn off when I had the desire to leave and bolt down a cheese pizza and a bag of chocolate drops before my name was called. I could eat, throw it back up, and be back in line within a half an hour.

I heard my name as I was heading for the door. As I trotted down the hallway, I noticed that the doors didn't have any names. They just had numbers. I had been told to open Door Number 2. If I was right, the grand prize was waiting.

A guy in a white coat was behind a desk. In front of it, there was one chair.

"Have a seat."

He didn't look up from his prescription pad. He was already signing one for me.

"What can I do for you?"

"Well, I'm worried about putting on too much weight. I've been a little stressed out lately, with exams and all. I start to eat and can't stop. Usually I'm not even hungry."

"Let's try this new combo drug to see if it will help. It's called Fen-Phen. It just became available and was designed to help the obese."

I was below my normal weight. Was that going to be a problem?

I kept quiet, and watched him sign the prescription. He handed it to me without looking up. He was already making out another one.

"You can get this filled at our own pharmacy here, if it's convenient. My receptionist can direct you. If you need a refill, just call and make an appointment. The law requires I see you personally, before I can refill it."

He hadn't seen me the first time. I walked back down the hall towards the waiting room with my magic script in my hand. I didn't have to ask where the pharmacy was; I just followed the anorectic herd when they left with their own prescriptions.

This was quite a lucrative operation for these doctors and the pharmacy. I figured the doctors were getting a kickback from the pharmacy on the $80.00 Fen-Phen bottle of 30 pills. At $60.00 a head, I calculated the diet clinic had made several hundred dollars in the hour I was there. Fine with me. I would have paid any price.

As I went to my car, I noticed the other girls and I were doing the same thing. Almost in unison, we uncapped our bottles of Fen-Phen, and each of us swallowed our first dose in the parking lot.

I could feel it working while I was driving back to the campus. It was exhilarating. I had found nirvana in a little brown bottle. I could almost see my heart thumping wildly inside my chest. I started to reach for my stash of candy in my glove compartment, and stopped. I had no appetite at all. I was ecstatic. This was better than the shot. It worked faster, and I had more of them. It was one of the happiest days of my addictive life. I was saved.

I would have called Mother right away, but she wouldn't remember why I called, anyway. Guess I'd have to celebrate all by myself. I was jumping all over the driver's seat. I reached out to turn the knob on the radio. I noticed my hand was shaking. Another positive sign. I found a rock station, and turned up the volume so loud it seemed the car was vibrating. I tapped my left foot along with the music, and pounded a beat on the steering wheel.

Damn, I LOVED this drug!

Chapter 7

My Love Affair

In the months I used Fen-Phen I was losing three pounds a week. My clothes were falling off of me. I bought low-cut blouses that showed off the top of my ribcage and collarbones. My face hollowed out. Empty skin hung from all parts of me. I considered cosmetic surgery to get rid of it. My parents didn't recognize me (they said proudly). I was on the ride of my life. This roller coaster was staying at the top and never coming down. I completed class assignments that weren't due for weeks. My roommate said I talked non-stop, and didn't sleep until I was exhausted. I'd get up after four hours, pop a pill and start all over again. I didn't need the bulimia everyday, like before. I had to force myself to eat. It was a fat girl's dream come true. I couldn't have been more pleased.

But it was a drug-induced high. I'd have to keep it going with the combo amphetamines. No problem. My diet doctor didn't even take my blood pressure or bother weighing me. Maybe that wasn't such a good idea.

The downside of this powerful combination was starting to make itself known. I lost so much fat my body began eating the muscle. I'd feel dizzy if I moved too fast. I had to use the banister on the stairs, or I could fall. Headaches became part of my morning when I'd awake after two to three hours of sleep. So I took more pills to offset the Fen-Phen. But I had a family history of addiction, and nobody had died yet. Besides, as I've said before about fat and death, it was a no-brainer. I would rather die than ever be fat again, and I didn't think twice about it. I wasn't really worried, though. I had the role model of the century, and she was still going. Both she and I had been doing this drug trip for quite a while now.

And after all was said and done, Mother and I were drug pros. She'd take tranquilizers to sleep at night, and stimulants to be able to function at work. If I swallowed enough 500 milligrams of Tylenol, I could get rid of the morning headaches. My liver is probably damaged from the overdoses of Tylenol.

I began to have a haunted expression, particularly around the eyes. They recessed from the skin that was losing its elasticity. I could hear my irregular heartbeat resonating through my ears. I became dehydrated from not taking in enough fluids. Kidney problems were becoming a certainty.

In addition to the negative physical changes, my personality altered and took a nosedive. I was impatient with everything. Time couldn't move fast enough for me. I'd have to jam my knees under the desk in front of me to keep from jumping up during the lectures. I couldn't keep my hands still. I had to make sure I wore something with pockets, even on the hottest days, so I could put my fists in them. I'd pinch the inside cloth between my knuckles, so my shaking hands were anchored there.

I was brusque with people. If they didn't talk at breakneck speed, I'd become bored. I'd finish their sentences for them, or walk away in the middle of a conversation. I was obsessed with my appearance. For someone who had avoided mirrors all her life, I found I couldn't get enough time in front of them. I was self-critical to the max. I had to see bone, or I'd be upset for the day. I knew exactly how many ribs I was supposed to be able to count, by looking at them in the mirror. If the count was off, I wouldn't eat for the next 24 hours. That was my time punishment. If my knee bones didn't hurt when I rubbed them together, I'd extend the 24 hours to 36 without food.

I'd point out the flaws in everyone. I was especially contemptuous of normal-sized people who didn't want to become thinner. They were too lazy or too stupid to diet. Fat girls got my harshest attention. I told any I ran into that if they couldn't keep from shoveling food down their throats, they should get their jaws wired. If I walked by a fat girl on campus, I'd mutter "Gross," so they would be sure to hear me. My years of self-hate turned into a righteous indignation whenever I saw fat girls. How could they live with themselves looking like that? The university should have a weight policy. Get thin or get out. What kind of careers would fat girls have, anyway? They were leeches on all of us who would have to support them. Maybe there were fat colleges where they could learn to become blue-collar workers. Certainly the white-collar world wouldn't have them. How would it look to have a fat girl in your office? Thin women wouldn't hire them, and men wouldn't want them. Males were only attracted to trophy girls who looked like models. Even if a fat girl was hired for an office job somewhere, she'd never get promoted. Anyone with any brains wouldn't be fat. Guess that summed up their mental ability.

I was relentless in my persecution of them. I started to seek them out. I called it "flushing them out" of the cafeteria and snack bars on campus. Weeknights, I'd make the rounds of the restaurants to find them. I'd sit down near them, and watch them while they ate. My disparaging stares and loud denunciations ran rampant for months.

I looked forward to my diet-den visits as the highlight of my week. I compared myself to those in the waiting room. If I wasn't thinner, I'd mentally beat myself up for hours.

My sister hadn't written for months. She lived in Tucson now, so we seldom saw each other, anyway. But I had been really critical of her in my last letters. I reminded her that she better not put on any extra pounds. People don't tolerate fat girls. Men wouldn't like her if she got fat. My letters were bitter and mean.

My parents avoided my phone calls. Mother refused to talk to me, after a vicious blow-up one weekend when I was home. I out-screamed her; I out-blamed her for every bad moment in my life. I told her she'd be better off dead than hanging around to inflict more damage on my father and me. I ran around the house to find her booze and pills. When I'd see some and raise them triumphantly above my head, Mother would try to grab them out of my hands. We almost came to blows. My father got between us.

"Don't talk to your mother that way."

"How can you defend her? Look at this stuff! She's a drug addict, and you know it."

"She's your mother. She deserves your respect, or you'll have to leave this house."

I glared at him.

"You never took my side. She's a nut case who ruined her life, and is destroying ours."

I balled up my fists at my sides, and moved threateningly towards the cause of all my troubles. She was the reason I got fat and had no friends when I was growing up. It had all started here – with her.

My father tried reason.

"You don't live here anymore. And your mother is a good woman."

Mother had attempted to shout me down. When her voice became hoarse, she began to cry.

I was pitiless. She had stolen my youth. I had to become her caretaker, when it should have been the other way around. All the years of emotional abuse came out in a rush of words. I suddenly realized I had become my mother.

I couldn't seem to stop myself from screaming at her. The Fen-Phen had my emotions revved up so high I couldn't seem to control myself.

"That's about enough."

My father had restrained me. As I struggled to free myself, he kept saying over and over again:

"What's wrong with you? Calm down."

Suddenly, I realized what I was doing. I stopped fighting against him. He took his arms away, and went to my mother. I stood there, exhausted and ashamed.

Good Lord, I had almost hit my mother.

I knew she was severely depressed and anxiety-ridden. She had overdosed on her pills several times. We thought she had forgotten how many she had taken. Maybe that hadn't been the case. When we had bailed her out of the drunk tank one Friday night, the officer said she had been going *up* the exit to the freeway, so she was driving into oncoming traffic. I chalked it up to her alcoholic intake. Perhaps she was suicidal. And I had just shouted into her face that she was better off dead.

I looked at her crumpled on the living room couch. My father had his arm around her. I couldn't believe it. I had done the same thing to her that her father had done for years. Only this time it was worse, because I knew what she had suffered.

I was in the throes of an emotional meltdown. And it was because of my magic pills I valued more than anything.

I looked at my father, and saw how much he loved her. I realized she had done the best she could under the circumstances. It was time to quit blaming her for what had happened in my life.

I went to the sliding glass doors.

"I'm sorry."

I couldn't tell them I was on drugs that had made this verbal assault take place. The irony was not lost on me.

The End of My Affair

Although I knew how potently dangerous Fen-Phen could be, I wasn't ready for the end of my love affair with it. Like the diet clinic that disappeared overnight, my Fen-Phen was gone just as abruptly. There were reports of heart valve damage from those taking the combo. Several girls had died.

I must say my first reaction was selfish. I needed it. I would take the risk. Life was better with it than without it. It was unfair to take it away from all of us, because a few anorectic girls had died. Big deal. They knew the risks. Nobody forced them to take the pills. Now all of us would suffer. Damn dumb bimbos. They couldn't even take their drug right. They were probably better off dead anyway. It just wasn't fair. Why give me this wonderful life and then take it away from me because some stupid worthless girls' hearts gave out. We knew we all were pretty much on a one-way trip as it was. We didn't expect to live a long life. But godammit, we deserved to enjoy the life we had because of our wonder drug. For most of us, it was the first time we could relax around food because we didn't want it. I knew my appetite would come back with a vengeance. The medical establishment could go to hell.

I was pretty dramatic about losing Fen-Phen. Addictions don't have emotional shades of gray; it's all or nothing. The body craves it on a physiological level. But it's wickedly bad on your mental state. Your brain made a special place for it. Now that area where your emotions live will be empty. And the drugs it has become addicted to permanently weren't going to be there to fill it.

It was terrible to lose my new best friend. The withdrawal from Fen-Phen was agonizing. It was mostly mental.

God, I'm going to have an appetite again.

I knew what would happen then. I wouldn't be able to control it. I'd eat everything in sight.

Naturally, I panicked.

Oh my God, I've lost my only friend.

Fen-Phen loved me. It gave me social acceptance and intimacy. The fat will come back. I'll be a social outcast again.

Wait a minute. Hold on a second. I have my trusty standby, I thought to myself. *My first love – my precious bulimia.*

I began that very day to renew my binge-and-purge ritual, with extra vigor. It had always given me what I really craved - affection. It would never desert me. I would make sure it couldn't be taken away from me. I could hide it - perfectly.

I let my OCD take over. I would be okay, until I could find another amphetamine drug fix.. I was intellectually gifted. I would do research. I'd reach my goal. I always had. If there were a way, I'd find it. I wouldn't stop until I did. Of course, that was my addicted brain talking. But I *had* to listen. My perfectionism would get me through this. I would not settle for less than an amphetamine equal to the one I couldn't have. It was only a matter of time until I found it. I systematically began to find a replacement for my beloved Fen-Phen.

Reading about Fen-Phen on the Internet was illuminating. It seemed the *combination* of the two drugs was dangerous, especially the Fenfluramine portion. Phentermine by itself didn't cause the heart valve tear. I just had to figure out how to get my phentermine back.

It wasn't going to be easy. The deaths had scared off even the diet doctors from prescribing any amphetamines at all. It was a "drug desert" for formerly fat girls for months.

The Internet rescued me. As I roamed around searching for articles on Fen-Phen, the online pharmacies latched onto me. They would provide as much phentermine as I wanted. It would be three times the price, and you couldn't be sure the pills didn't contain rat poison. There were no guarantees. I didn't care. I needed my diet-drug fix. And there were hundreds of sites that offered me the affection I was missing. My two addictions could co-exist again. Salvation was a keystroke away.

You had to avoid the legitimate sites that wanted a doctor's prescription. The FDA was on the trail of drugs purchased on the Internet, and shipped in from other countries. It could be hazardous to order them, and have them traced back to you. If they did intercept your order, they sent you a notice. You could leave the drug with them to destroy, and it would go no farther.

I could live with that. I discovered you could order from several online pharmacies at the same time. If they weren't connected by one outsource or warehouse which shipped for several pharmacies, you could take the risk of losing a bottle now and then to the FDA.

Even 'though I had resumed my binge-and-purge routine at an increased pace to stave off the weight, I had the awful feeling the fat cells were still filling and pushing into the empty skin I treasured so much. I was vomiting after every meal in addition to the binges and purges. My stomach hurt, my breath constantly smelled of vomit, and I was miserable all the time. I couldn't even get interested to sex. Everything but the bulimia fell by the wayside. For the first time in my life, I didn't care about my grades, and it showed. When I was headed for academic probation, I ate enough to give me the energy to do my assignments and attend my classes. I lived for the school holidays so I could sleep all day. I was totally strung out and exhausted at the same time.

I went to every health store in town, looking for a replacement. Nothing worked. I just had diarrhea all the time when I used whatever I found that said "diet" on their shelves.

Of course, it didn't help when I would triple the amount of pills I was supposed to take. The only thing I got that worked was the water pills. I peed away about five pounds, but I was constantly dehydrated.

I started to cut myself to ease the pain. I had slivers of red welts down both arms on the insides. I couldn't go anywhere without a long-sleeved shirt or sweater, or people would stare at the angry blood-red gouges. Some of them became infected. Pus stained the clothing covering them. I probably became septic at some point, but I didn't give a shit. Oh, and I couldn't do that either – no bowel movements. My stomach looked distended. I'd sit on the commode for hours, but nothing happened. My life sucked.

Not only the mental and physical effects were a nuisance, but it was a lot more bother to use the bulimia by itself. It was getting to the point I had to store my stomach contents in jelly jars until I could load them into my backpack, and take them to the big garbage cans behind the restaurants surrounding the campus.

I couldn't go to the same bins, either. There was always the risk a restaurant employee would come out to empty the restaurant leftovers, and catch me in the process of pouring out the jars.

I also had to keep the jars instead of throwing them away with the vomit. It was too hard to buy them, eat all the jelly, use them, and buy new ones. I cleaned them thoroughly, but sometimes I would retch when I'd see the globs of upchucked food attached to the sides and bottom. I used a toothbrush to scrub in the deepest part of the jars.

With so much eating, regurgitating, and getting rid of the evidence, I was spending most of my days occupied with my bulimia. I was more tired than usual after I had purged. Since it was so often, my throat was raw in places. If I wasn't careful because I was usually in a hurry, I could jam my nails into the back of my throat instead of down it. I'd know I'd snagged some skin at the back of my throat when I spit up blood with the vomit. I cut my nails to the quick so it would be harder for them to catch on any tissue as I thrust them down my throat.

I was so depleted after I upchucked, I would lean on the edge of the toilet and gasp with my mouth open like a fish tossed on the grass to die. Because I lost track of the time, often there was just enough time to use the toilet paper to sop up the glob dripping from my vomit arm before I had to get out of the bathroom if my roommate came back to our room. I'd hurry to get the essentials done before I would nonchalantly open the bathroom door to chat with her.

I knew that I needed to run the toilet paper through each of my vomit fingers. I'd so it as quickly as possible in the sink. I'd have the water running, so any leftover from the toilet paper could go down the drain. If she came and went, I could begin the bulimic bathroom-cleaning process.

Fortunately, my roommate was out most of the time. And when she did return from a date, she'd only change her clothes and leave. She had come to the university to party. She'd probably get her degree in about six years. Fine with me. I had privacy and my bulimic rituals.

I could take my time in my locked bathroom at home. Here at the dorm, my roommate could come in anytime, and want to use our bathroom. I tried to schedule my bulimic activity in my dorm room when she had classes, or was on a date. Still, if her class was canceled or she had forgotten something, I couldn't be stuffing my face from my food pile on the floor or bent over the toilet, in case she came back early or unexpectedly.

I needed my upper. It worked beautifully with my other addiction. It was time to test the waters, and order phentermine on the Internet.

My Ship Comes In

When I first cruised the Internet for my drug of choice, I had to wait until my roommate was gone before I could look at the various Internet drug sites. Finally, she left for a date. If she liked the guy, I wouldn't see her till morning. She'd sneak back in when the doors were opened at 7. I just had to yell "All present," when the head resident did bed checks.

I found a couple of sites that looked good, and didn't need a doctor's prescription. They asked some questions about my health. I checked a box at the bottom that absolved them of any liability. This was familiar territory so far. I had a choice of strength and number. I wanted the 37.5 milligrams, the strongest, and three-months' worth. It had been three weeks since my last Fen-Phen, so I was eager to get the amphetamine back in my system. I chose the Overnight shipping. It cost an extra $28.00, but that was the least of my worries. I needed my comfort drug as soon as possible.

It took two days to get my first bottle. The pharmacy made you sign for it. The signature probably protected them from prosecution in some way. They didn't ask for identification, though, when they required you to sign for it. Bonzo the Clown could say he was me, and the guy would put it in his hands.

The intercom in my room buzzed.

"You've got a package. You've got to sign for it."

I felt like singing "Happy Days Are Here Again," as I almost flew down the stairs to the foyer to get my first shipment of phentermine.

The Fed-Ex guy handed me a relatively flat and light package. It had a small bump where the pill container was. He gave me a clipboard, and I signed on the line next to my name.

I was tempted to open it right there, but if the girl behind the desk was watching, it would be a tad difficult to explain a bottle full of blue pills that didn't resemble vitamins one bit. I *was* doing something illegal.

The white package was stamped with lots of foreign stamps. I really didn't care which Third World country had provided me with my drug. It was what was in the package that counted.

When I got back to my room, I closed and locked the door behind me. The package had a strip you could pull to open it. I tugged, and it came away cleanly with a little ripping sound. My senses seemed to be heightened already in anticipation of what I would soon feel inside again.

The small brown pharmacy bottle dropped into my hand as I upended the mail envelope. I held the bottle for an instant. I enjoyed the feel of it. I revolved it in my hand. My fingers traced the typing on the white sticker. I closed my eyes. I waited as long as I could before opening them and reading the label. I didn't recognize the doctor's name. It looked Indian. It said the dosage was 37.5. If you went to a regular doctor who prescribed Phentermine, you had to start with the lowest dose. Another advantage of using the online pharmacies.

I made a bell shape of my fingers and lowered them to the cap. As I unscrewed the lid, my heart began beating like the drug had already jolted it. When I looked inside, a mound of small, oblong, blue, gelatin capsules lay in a heap from the bottom to the middle of the bottle. I tipped the bottle, so that one of the capsules rolled into my hand. I could see *phentermine* and *37.5* stamped on the sides of the pill. These must be the real thing. No imitations. It must be so, because the name is spelled correctly. Only a certified pharmacist would be sure to have pills with correct spelling.

Wait a second.

How hard is it to make a stamp with the name of the amphetamine correctly spelled? I think I just wanted to believe these were true pharmaceutical products. It didn't seem like such a bad thing, then, to get them like this. Instead of paying for a doctor's visit and then getting a prescription, I could get it directly from the source. Whatever and wherever that was. Hopefully, it was not some dirty bathtub mixture that unwashed hands scooped into these little brown bottles. I had a vivid imagination, as a well as a good memory of cop programs on television that featured how illegal drugs were made.

This was exciting. I guess it was because it was forbidden, and I had fantasized about having the pill physically in my hand. My right hand was my bulimic hand, so I would use my left hand to deliver the amphetamine. I would put it between the first two fingers of my left hand. I would place the torpedo-shaped capsule as far back on my tongue as I could reach without setting off the gag reflect. This was one time when I wouldn't welcome that particular help. The blue capsule would slide down faster. The gelatin covering would begin to melt. It would break open. The crystals would invade my bloodstream. My brain was ready and waiting for the rush of chemicals to reach it.

It seems I was attracted to the rituals as much as the addictive behaviors. Maybe my perfectionism needed each step of the process to be done slowly and thoroughly. It was certainly exhilarating to complete the final steps.

I sat on the edge of my bed. I waited for the charge amphetamines gave me. It was like getting a body shock from electrodes hooked up to a battery. This one wasn't as powerful as the Fen-Phen's kick, but I could immediately tell something was happening.

I got up, went into the bathroom, and looked at my face in the mirror above the sink. My skin was starting to flush. My eyes were beginning to dilate. My hands holding the edge of the sink began to tremble. And the final moment of truth. I put my left hand on my heart. I could feel it beating faster. It was working.

I went back to my bed, picked up the bottle and hid it in a zippered part of my purse. Contentedly, I patted it like I would a child who had performed well.

I turned off the light, and sat down at my desk. My hands were starting to shake a bit more now. I knew I wouldn't be able to sleep. Might as well have a food party. It seemed right to binge and purge with the amphetamine racing through my body and brain. It was like saying hello to old friends who were together again. I was relieved and contented.

For the remainder of my last year in college, I got my overseas drug on a regular basis. My phentermine package would arrive at least once a week. Sometimes, I'd get two deliveries. They would have different foreign stamps on them. The doctors' names on the label would never be the same. I tried not to use the same pharmacy twice. I thought it would make me less likely to attract attention on the Internet, or from the authorities. Since there were so many online pharmacies, it wasn't hard to find a new one every week. After a month, I started getting e-mails from all kinds of overseas pharmacies. They probably had a database and automatically sent out drug bulletins to frequent buyers. Everything is tracked nowadays.

My parents had put plenty of school money on my credit card. That kept me from coming home on a regular basis to ask for more. Maybe I'm being too cynical here. No, I don't think so, now that I think about it. Anyway, I saved money by borrowing textbooks, so I could spend my book funds on junk food and phentermine.

I was used to allocating my weekly allowance for buying my comfort food. My parents didn't ask me to account for the $20.00 they gave me each week. Maybe they thought I was going to the movies, or buying books to read. As long as I wasn't causing them problems, I could pretty much do as I liked.

Okay, so I had a good cache of the drug. Even if the unimaginable happened and I couldn't get any right away, I'd be fine. I felt like a chipmunk that had stored enough nuts to last through the winter. Frequently after a binge, I'd pop one of my little blue darlings. It would get rid of the physical exhaustion the bulimia caused. I had the world in the palm of my hand – either a cupcake or a phentermine. When I'd get too jumpy to study, I'd go for a walk until the dorm closed its doors. If I really was on edge, I'd hit one of the bars and dance until my legs ached. My startle reflex kept me from snagging guys for sex. The only down side to my best friend.

My senses were wired, too. I could smell everything. From the cologne on my various dance partners to the cigarette residue on their shirts,even if we weren't close on the dance floor. My perfume mixed with whatever cologne they had on. Sometimes it was the odor of a man's sweat or the liquor he had on his lips as I leaned in to listen to him talk in the crowded, music-deafening atmosphere.

I was tempted to go home with many of them but realized I'd be too much on the phentermine high to enjoy sex. Since I could feel and taste at a higher level than anyone else, it was enough to rub against them in the bars and catch a few goodbye kisses as I left to make it back to the dorm before curfew. My mind would race so fast, I often forgot what the last one looked like or said before I moved on to the next. When I didn't force myself to study or get papers done for classes in my room, bar-hopping was my favorite pastime.

Fat Girls Never Have Fun

During the final month before graduation, recruiters came to the campus quite often. It was a prestigious university, so its graduates were highly sought after. I was hired after my first interview. I got a contract in the mail several weeks after the recruiter had left. Since I was graduating with honors and was incredibly slim, I had no doubts I would get the job.

It was in Hawaii. I committed for two years. My parents, who had forgiven my outburst, were proud of what I had accomplished or perhaps it was the stick figure they finally had for their oldest daughter. Mother bragged at work about her fashionably thin, college-grad daughter getting her first job in Honolulu, Hawaii. My father congratulated me and shook my hand at graduation. He said to send postcards.

The flight was long, but they had lots of movies, television programs or pre-recorded music you could plug into. And it was before they stopped serving so many meals, so we could eat something every hour if we wanted. I had taken a phentermine in the airport restroom before I boarded the plane. I just nibbled at the food in the square trays put continually in front of me.

In the middle of the flight, I could feel the urge to eat, so I took another blue pill to make it the rest of the way without gorging. I didn't think I could purge in the tiny plane bathrooms. It wasn't because of their size necessarily. I was like a twig. When I got up to walk back to the bathrooms in Coach, my hips wouldn't get near the seats on either side. I could casually make my way down the long corridor. No problem.

I was afraid to binge because the plane was full. The restrooms were in constant use. I could probably have vomited in the allotted time people spend in the little rooms, but I couldn't be sure someone wouldn't be waiting outside. Even 'though the engines were incredibly noisy, I didn't know if the sound of my retching could be heard through the restroom doors. They looked thick enough. I didn't want to risk it, 'though. It was definitely a struggle not to binge and purge. My routine was being disrupted. I hoped my fat cells were being occupied with the amphetamine coursing through the blood surrounding them.

For the final leg of the trip, I didn't eat anything. I had to drink water so I wouldn't get dehydrated and develop leg cramps. But other than a small plastic cup of water, I was food-chaste. The second phentermine was doing the trick.

When we arrived, I got my overnight bag from the storage bin above my head, and waited for the passengers to be allowed to disembark. I could hear Hawaiian music coming from outside the plane. As I bent down and looked out the small plane windows, I saw a brightly painted bus pull up to the gangway. It had speakers attached to all sides. They were blaring Don Ho's *Tiny Bubbles* for all they were worth.

By the way, after two years of hearing that song everywhere I went, I developed a strong dislike for it. *Bland* would be a kind way to describe it.

We boarded the loud bus, with its colors and music assaulting the senses, and headed for the terminal. The ride seemed to take as long as the flight. Evidently, the leisurely rhythm of Ho's song was indicative of the pace of everything on the island.

Men in white pants and neon-colored shirts, and women in faux-straw skirts and bold pink-shaded tops were waiting to wish us "Aloha," and put a string of scented flowers around our necks. I thought the leis were beautiful and smelled great. The band standing next to them playing (you guessed it) *Tiny Bubbles* I could have done without. The matrons in their polyester pantsuits loved it, 'though.

Just a side note here. Fat females should not wear form-fitting outfits in eye-squinting colors that make their bodies look like ship bulkheads. I hadn't eaten, so the sight of those mammoth behinds jiggling to a song with the word *tiny* in it was enough to make me quite queasy. I didn't want to *even* get into the bubble butt comparison. *Superiority* was my thin middle name. I didn't even have to stretch my highly educated brain to come up with fat jokes. It was too easy. I headed off to get my luggage.

After I had retrieved my bags, I searched for the city bus to take me into town. I had reserved a room at the YWCA until I could find an apartment to share.

Since I was so skinny, I could put my two big bags on the bus seat with me.

Smugly, I looked at the different sizes of people outside the airport bus, as we passed them on the way to the local hotels and, in my case, the YWCA. Men with beer bellies and women with fat legs ending with chubby toes in throng-footwear were moving like whale pods down the beach sidewalk.

Fat girls who tried to emulate the slender female Hawaiian dancers had tops and bottoms made of cloth that barely covered them. Tight bodices had massive flesh overflowing like ugly putty. The small bottom part of the outfit did little to cover the sea of cellulite rolling across their legs. I was definitely feeling sick to my stomach again. This was not the vacation spot for obese tourists.

I felt the need for another phentermine, but I couldn't get into my purse. It was wedged between my two oversized bags. The *only* thing oversized about me, I might add.

I would discover Hawaii was a particularly terrible place for fat girls. For starters, the fancy beach hotels didn't want them around. The locals selling fake necklaces and bracelets had nothing big enough to fit them, so they were unprofitable, extra-large obstacles on the beach that were in the way of slender rich tourists. Apartment owners saw them as grotesque slabs, taking up the whole beach and bringing down property values.

Arrogantly, I could mentally tic off multitudinous reasons the islands didn't welcome fat girls with open arms. The natives didn't want to open their arms to them at all, much less put leis around their necks, as the fat haoles ("strangers" in Hawaiian, which became "whites," a derogatory term) clumsily rotated their huge bodies off their planes.

Leis were made of expensive flowers. Fat girls needed big leis. Nobody wanted to get that close to put one on, either. It would look like trying to throw a ring around an enormous misshapen object at a carnival from twenty feet away. It was not the image the public relations folks wanted to encourage.

Then, there's that entire span of glaring white sand with bunches of cellulite-free females in their 20s lying around in those bathing suits made for dolls. There weren't enough beach umbrellas or mammoth towels in the entire state to cover the deep cellulite pits on fat girls' bodies. The backs of their legs looked like exploded mine fields.

They have muumuus in Hawaii, comfortable cloth dresses that easily slip over your head. But they were not originally designed to cover the bulbous shapes of abundantly flesh-packed girls visiting the tropical isles. The expensive stores would disdainfully regard fat girls with indifference, if not outright hostility, if it appeared a fat girl was thinking about entering their store. So they put their pricey, mute-colored pastel muumuus on wafer-thin mannequins in their display windows. Just to show they had no muumuus for gargantuan female figures.

But since these are dresses without any shape, so you can be as rotund as you want and still find something to wear, fat girls embraced them like lovers. The beachfront tourist places had hundreds of cheap ones. They were probably made in factories by fat girls who couldn't use regular sewing machines because of their thick fingers. The stitching was minimal. Down one side and up the other.

Of course the patterns on the inexpensive ones were awful. Tons of huge flowers in the brightest colors imaginable. A fat girl wearing a muumuu was like a parade float waddling down the sidewalk. Heaven forbid she stepped off into sand. It would take a tow truck to suck her out. All the tanning, pretty people would use her for entertainment as she struggled to keep her muumuu down, while several really strong men formed a human chain to pull her out. It would be the one time the beach bodybuilders would notice her. These Adonises would think of her as another weight apparatus. They would flex their enormous muscles as the bikini-waifs, lying barely on top of the sand, formed admiring "Os" with their raspberry-flavored, lip-balmed mouths.

Fat girls in muumuus are absolutely grotesque (I was so self-righteous in my thinness). Even the most spacious dresses struggled to cover fat-girl legs. Mounds of calves and ankles would appear in front of normal people when the slender folks were taking leisurely strolls down the sandy walkways. Following a fat girl in a muumuu, was not part of the perfect picture of an island vacation. It was enough to put you off your mahi-mahi.

"Let's go around her."

"How many days do we have left of our vacation? It'll take at least three to get all the way around."

The vacationers would smirk, and laugh out loud. The fat girl would hear everything. She knew better than to bend over to pick up seashells.

When my first day as a thin in Honolulu ended with a barefoot walk down the beach, I would feel my beautiful space was invaded if a fat girl appeared in my line of vision. The images were definitely anti-paradisiacal. The deep indentations of their fat toes in the sand. Their voluminous dresses pulled up by the breezes coming in off the turquoise water, to show mountains of fat fighting for territory on the backs of their thighs and knees. Their bending over to pick up seashells would look like mutated giant squids tangled in seaweed. Fat girls lost their balance easily when they changed their upright position for another. My lip would curl when I saw them fall over into the surf, like hot air balloons semi-inflated. Ugly to the max.

No wonder even the rapacious local sellers didn't sell food around them on the beach. The venders who sold local cuisine wouldn't get near them. Who'd want to buy something, and then feel like upchucking when they saw a fat girl eating the same thing?

The only use for fat girls would be as living sand dumps. Kids could play king-of-the-mountain or pirate games on them. If a fat girl didn't make a movement to show she was alive, children would bury her in wet sand and carve trenches. Well, at least the fat girls would have a purpose. And they would be covered up. The only saving grace to them being on the beach with the rest of us. To keep the kids occupied.

As I watched Waikiki pass by, I promised myself I wouldn't ever return to being a human sand dune. I would never relapse. I would be one of the herds of beach bunnies soaking up the rays. I would have the non-gay bodybuilders lasciviously eyeing my body like I was a twenty-dollar steak. I would have so much sex I would walk bow-legged for weeks. The Hawaiian public relations firms could hire me as a living brochure for the beauty of the island.

While I was fantasizing about my future, I was also looking for a place to rent. The YWCA was fine for a couple of days, but living out of a suitcase can get old fast. I'd take the local paper with me to the beach early in the morning. Usually, there were some surfers riding the waves. There would be some beach umbrellas tied up and stored against the low wall that was built along the resort beaches. I'd grab one of the big umbrellas, set it up, and peruse the paper and the surfers. All was right with my world. I was thin; I was in.

Then, I moved into an apartment with a fat girl. It was the worst thing that could have happened to me. My slim college figure started to go.

When you live with someone fat, you can eat more because you know you're not as fat as she is. I didn't start with the muumuu dresses, but I ended up there. I traded the food for the phentermine and bulimia. I was always going to be thinner than the girl I was living with. I could let go of my addictions in the land of sun and fun. Besides, it was too much trouble to secretly purge. I could binge all I wanted without any consequences I could see. It helped that I covered up everything with ever-bigger clothing, so I *couldn't* see the fat landing like a 747 all over me. *Overeaters Anonymous* didn't exist in my vocabulary.

As is often the case with addictive personalities, I had programmed my brain to expect certain stimuli. If it wasn't going to be satiated with bulimia and amphetamines, it would take hold of the next addiction to come its way. I became a foodaholic. Eating pacified me, as usual. But now I didn't care if the food stayed where it was. I let my stomach expand to accommodate the vast amounts of stuff coming its way every hour. There was no one to judge me. My roommate ate more than I did. I went from self-critical to self-oblivious. I didn't bother with rationalizations. I just ate, and kept on eating.

Just in case I *might* be allowing too much weight to descend on me, I'd put the first two fingers on my formerly bulimic right hand around the wrist of the other. It was my caliper-measuring *modus operandi*. If I could easily get my fingers around, then I wasn't fat. That's not the place I should have been measuring.

My heavyweight roommate had never dieted. She seemed happy the way she was. Maybe her whole family was fat, so she didn't know any different. When I found out she was from Texas, that explained a lot. Wasn't everything huge in Texas?

Chapter 8

Work World

My first job brought out the personality traits Mother had given me. Her formative background echoed resoundingly in my work behavior. My engrained "people pleaser" persona was a result of Mother's unfortunate history. It would play a major part in the evolution of my addictive behavior.

From the local Business College where she was the top student in her Shorthand class, to her job as a secretary after she married my father and had me, Mother was a typical woman of her period. She was passive and submissive with people, especially male authority figures. Women had come from the age when "A woman's place was in the home", to second-class members of society that were allowed to work to support the family income. Mother's natural intelligence had been suppressed by a 50s society that relegated her to helpmate in the home and assistant in the workplace.

Her father's generation had been particularly strict about a woman's place in a man's world. My stepmother was never allowed to work outside the home. My father ran the store by himself, with paid help from local boys in the neighborhood. Mother would work in the back room, keeping track of the inventory and candling eggs. Her father kept the books, of course. She wasn't trusted with the higher thinking skills involved with the store's accounts. Neither Mother nor her stepmother knew what the family income was. The "breadwinner" role was the man's alone. A bright talented woman like Mother accepted her role, but inwardly resented it. There was no outward show of rebellion, especially in her home. Her submissive behavior with her father was augmented by his dictatorial demeanor and mood swings. His alcoholism and depression were hidden. She just thought she was never good enough.

In one of her storytelling episodes with me later, she said her father wished she had died instead of her mother. He hadn't wanted children, anyway. And then look what happened.

To survive in her repressive home environment, Mother became the consummate "people pleaser" in every phase of her life. Her life-long anxiety and deep depression fed her low self-image. The words "I'm sorry" were out of her mouth before anything had occurred in her business classes and in her home.

She had the singing voice to make it in the world. People loved her voice. When she became a bitter alcoholic, she would drunkenly rail against her father and us because she had never had the chance to sing professionally.

Although her parents had been dead for many years, she was still suffering the effects of her father's mistreatment. Her stepmother's passivity didn't help. Of course, living with an alcoholic was like walking an emotional tightrope. She learned later after her father had died, that her stepmother probably had to quietly battle with him. Confrontation could be dangerous. But at the time her father was disciplining her, it probably looked to her like she was alone.

I think Mother was afraid to try to pursue a singing career. What if she failed? It was a tough world to compete in. Just because she was a star in high school and church, didn't mean she had any real talent. What if someone didn't like her singing? She was so self-critical and fearful of rejection she wouldn't put herself out there. She never fought for herself. People wouldn't like it if she had opinions of her own. She was probably smarter than the people she worked with *and* her boss. But she couldn't show it. They wouldn't like that. They wouldn't love her.

I think she fought those demons in herself the rest of her life. She used alcohol to disguise the pain she felt everyday, when she went into work with her obligatory smile and cookies. Her alcoholism and subsequent prescription drug abuse would most likely eventually kill her. It looked like I was on the same path. My first foray into the work world turned out to be the ideal place to start.

I "people pleased" all over the place. I was so afraid my colleagues wouldn't like me I smiled like a damn idiot at them all the time.

One day when I was in the bathroom sitting on the toilet, the sliding latch on the stall door came loose. A woman came in, saw the opening door, and started to come in. She was surprised to find me on the commode. I was so submissive I smiled at her and almost said I was sorry for being in there. You should be here instead of me. That was about as low as you can go in self-esteem. I was my mother's daughter, for sure.

When I got heavy and began wearing muumuus to work, I was scared to death they would think I was getting fat. I didn't eat lunch or any of the treats people brought in. I bought hundreds of dollars worth of candy for them during the years I was there. I smoked to cut my appetite at work. I had used up the phentermine I had brought with me in the first few months. I had popped one in my mouth whenever I had needed an energy boost. I didn't use it to control my weight anymore, so I didn't order more.

I didn't want my peers to think I was a pig, a human eating machine, a fat slob at work. Appearance was everything.

When I got back to the apartment, though, I wasn't concerned about what my roommate saw me eat. She was eating right along with me. She wasn't one of the thins I had to do anything for, to get approval and affection. Anything – like letting the toilet door keep opening when a colleague pushed on it when I was on the toilet.

I was thinner than my roommate. That was the rationale I used, to let myself go with my food addiction. It was the fat-girl denial of what was real. And I was a perfect foodaholic; a determined food addict - as good as I was a bulimic and phentermine user. I didn't want to see the irony.

I took to my new life with vigor. And I had willing company for the first time.

Eating Everything But the Box

We would get home from work with ravenous appetites. Nothing was safe if it was edible. We would eat entire boxes of spaghetti dinners for four by ourselves, one box for each of us. We bought the heftiest cans of Parmesan cheese to smother the reams of spaghetti. On the weekends, we'd go to the drive-in movies with the back seat full of snacks and sodas.

After a couple of months, I noticed the clothes I had brought with me from the mainland were getting awfully tight. Well, that's not a problem in Hawaii. The local muumuu stores number in the hundreds. Tourists love to bring the cheap, neon-colored sack dresses back for their aunts, fat sisters, and grandmothers. It was like an ocean of colored cloth just waiting for me. I dove right in after my suit pants ripped in the crotch while I was sitting at my desk one day. The fat bulged through like enormous amounts of bread dough. It was massively white and spongy. I tried stapling the rip, but the fat burst out in other places at the same time I was squeezing the first place shut. Safety pins worked, until I could get in my rented car to go back to the apartment. That day I shopped for my first muumuu and never looked back.

At the end of my first year in Hawaii, my roommate had to go back stateside, so I was left to happily become obese on my own. Now, I could eat and throw the wrappers on the floor. I could leave the dishes in the sink until I ran out, and was forced to wash them. Since it was a nuisance to waste time cooking, I would pick up fast food on my way home from work, and binge from the time I stepped through the door with my junk food until I went to sleep at night.

I did notice that it was getting more and more difficult to sleep in any position but on my side. I was probably snoring, too. Sleep apnea is common with obesity.

The bed was king-sized. I could convince myself that I wasn't too fat, because there was still plenty of space on the bed when I laid down. I didn't want to notice that the space was getting smaller and smaller as the weeks of binge eating went on.

Along with the bed, the apartment had a huge tub in the bathroom. When I had first seen the overlarge deep bathtub when I had initially moved in, I was elated. I usually took showers. Mother had found it disgusting to think that people would sit in their own dirt in a bathtub, so our bathtub remained pristine because it was never used. I had always wondered what it would be like to float in warm water, with gigantic bubbles coating your whole body. Now, I would get the chance in the apartment in Hawaii

Once in a while, I would indulge in a bubble bath. But the last time I took one with no one in the apartment, I had trouble getting out of the tub. I chalked it up to slippery tub sides from the colored sprinkles that had become multi-colored, scented bubbles. It took more and more bubble sprinkles to make bubbles to completely cover me in the tub. My final session in the bubble bath ended in disaster for the shower curtain and towel rack. I had tried to use both to get some leverage to pull myself up, so I could step over the lip of the tub. They both came loose from the wall.

The damage did have a quasi-positive side to it. After I got dressed, I called the landlord to tell him about the bathroom fixtures coming away from the wall. Since it was probably the only time that had happened in one of his units, he was pretty curious about how it had happened. I had my story all ready.

"I called the cable company to come out and fix the signal yesterday. The cable guy said that he had to use the bathroom, so I told him to go ahead. I was in the back room when I heard a loud noise coming from the bathroom. I knocked on the door. He answered and said that he had put his tool case on the shower curtain, and he had rested his arm on the towel rack while he was using the facilities. When the weight of the tool case made it start to slip off the shower curtain, he made a grab for it, and got tangled in the curtain as he tried to catch it. He had held onto the towel rack, so he wouldn't fall forward as he was reaching for the tool kit before it could drop and dent the floor. Well, everything came loose. He was really embarrassed about everything, and didn't charge us for the cable connection he had to fix."

I thought the last bit might do the trick, since cable repair was one of the most expensive things that could happen in an apartment. Definitely more than putting a new shower rod and towel rack in.

I held my breath.

"Okay, I understand. I'll have someone come and look at it today. Will you be home this afternoon?"

Of course, I would, since I stayed in the apartment eating until I went to bed.

"Yes, I'll be here after 3:30."

"Fine then. I'll send him this afternoon."

Since food had replaced sex, I hadn't really missed my sexual binges. But there in my doorway, waiting to come in to fix my bathroom, was one of those coppertone Hawaiian males that look good enough to eat in those commercials advertising the wonders of the islands. All of a sudden, I felt urges I had forgotten existed.

He showed me his identification, and walked right into an erotic fantasy I had while he was replacing the rod and rack in the bathroom.

I would come in the bathroom to see if he needed anything. I would be wearing a muumuu I could pull down off my shoulders to show the deep cleft between my big breasts. He would turn, and I'd bump into his chest. I'd have to hold onto him to keep my balance. He would grab me by my uncovered shoulders to make sure I didn't fall. I'd look him in the eye while I moved his hand from my shoulder to my breast. He would look surprised for an instant, and try to pull his hand away. I'd capture it and press it against the hard nipple showing through the thin cloth. He would glance down, and then back up into my eyes. I'd give him a hot look and moan a little, while I kept pushing his hand into my heavy white globe that had popped out of the now-falling muumuu. He would bring me closer to him with his other hand, and we would kiss, his lips crushing mine.

As I pulled him out of the bathroom and down the hall with my lips still attached to his, I'd start to unbutton his brown work shirt, while his hands were now both gripping my buttocks, kneading the flesh and bringing a rosy tint to the surface. His shirt would drop to the floor. I didn't want those big heavy hands of his to move, so I quickly unbuckled his belt, pulled down his zipper, and his pants fell to the bedroom carpet.

"Was that all you needed, ma'am?"

I was snapped out of my reverie by his voice. At first, I thought he was talking about sex. But no, he was asking me, fully clothed with his nametag undisturbed on his shirt pocket, whether I had anything else for him to do.

I hesitated before I answered. Would he?

He had turned away to take out his job slip for me to sign.

"No, thank you. That will be it." I closed the door behind him, went to my bedroom, and had sex with the bed blanket.

Well, if sex with a man was out of the question, then I could still indulge in my favorite outdoor pastime – sunbathing. Of course, there was a slight catch since I had put on so much weight.

Ironically, although I have always taken the opportunity to enjoy the sun whenever I could, I couldn't do it in a place with beaches that were celebrated for it. The thins were there. So on weekends, I'd put on my one-piece bathing suit, and take the elevator to the apartment roof, where I could put two deck chairs together to make a sort of plastic lounge. I had purchased extra-large beach towels to go along with the muumuus. The ones I had in the apartment no longer fit when I got out of the shower. Hawaii has thousands of expansive, flower-covered beach towels for sale. The tourists like them as much as the muumuus.

I'd wrap a big towel around my middle, and make for the elevator. I 'd hope the elevator would be empty, because the elastic in my suit would be cutting into my upper thighs, and I had to keep pulling it down. When there were people in the elevator, they were surprised when I pushed the roof button. Most people in bathing suits and towels would be heading down to the beach. I had seen what happened to fat girls on the beach at Waikiki. It wasn't pretty.

I'd be trying to hide in the back of the elevator, just in case someone came in at one of the floors. Sometimes that damn ding would ring, and it would stop at a floor.

The elevator doors would open. The waiting apartment resident would regard me in a quandary.

"Are you going up?"

"Yes."

"Is there a pool on the roof?"

"No."

"Oh, then, I guess I'll wait for the next one going down."

Worse yet, some of them would ride up with me if they didn't want to wait. I tried to look as nonchalant as possible in my multi-colored beachwear. But I raged inside at the slowness of the elevator, and was perpetually worried the other occupants would want to chat with me about the roof.

When the doors opened onto the roof, they would peer out for a moment, thinking that maybe there was a sundeck up there they hadn't known about. I'd push through to the opening. My hips bumped anyone standing in front of me like bumper cars. I was frantically holding onto the towel around my waist with one hand, and suntan oil, book, hat, and sunglasses in the other. I knew if the towel started slipping, to hell with whatever I was holding in the other hand. Keeping that towel up was my first priority.

"Excuse me."

Oh, no. Oh my God.

One thigh was starting to show, as I moved as quickly as I could to the opening doors. As I maneuvered to cover myself, I'd usually drop something. If I bent over to pick it up, I knew I was lost. My butt would hit whoever was behind me, and I'd probably drop everything else.

"Did you drop this?"

"Yes, thanks."

Clutching everything as if my life depended on it, I lumbered out the door, and made my way to the two upright deck chairs I turned into a long plastic bed. I'd put the towel on the chairs after I pulled them together. After putting on my hat, sunglasses and suntan oil, I'd begin to read the trashy romance novel I'd brought.

The plots were all the same. Some skinny girl getting the muscled man of her dreams. Hell, even the romance novels were against me. Evidently, fat girls didn't get princes in shining armor.

There were no fat girls in the novels, unless they were cooks or housekeepers. They were referred to as being pleasantly plump, motherly types with fourteen-children-sagging breasts, who frequently hugged the heroine during her token sad moments, before her life turned out just as she wanted it to. I guess romance-novel writers knew no one would publish a book about fat girls falling in love. Fat girls didn't get love, because they were too busy eating anything that moved.

If I fell asleep, I wouldn't notice the deck chairs slowly separating from the weight of my thighs and calves. I'd awaken abruptly to find me hanging between the two chairs, my arms clutching the chair arms that were slick from the suntan oil. Kicking my legs to pull the other chair towards me was a reflex action that usually didn't work. I'd land with an audible thump on the hot pavement. Fortunately, the towel was buried underneath, so I didn't get burned when I landed sprawled on my back. It was anything but graceful. My legs and arms frantically tried to find something to latch onto. I must have looked like one of those enormous dinosaurs with the tiny arms.

Yuck.

"What is that, mommy?"

"We mustn't stare, sweetheart. It's probably some poor animal that has fallen, and can't get up."

"Can we help it?"

"No, dear, sometimes it's just their time to go."

The Plane or You

When I had been to the islands for two years, the money I was earning couldn't keep up with the inflated prices increasing each year. Whatever I had left over after paying the rent of the apartment and car went to food. That wasn't something I wanted to dwell on. It wasn't because I was embarrassed about buying so much food. It was the fact that I didn't have enough money left to get all the eats I wanted.

It was time to go home. I maxed out my credit card for a ticket back to the mainland.

The flight was long again, so I loaded up on candy at the discount market before I arrived at the airport and turned in my rental car. I stowed away the four 1-lb. bags in my voluminous purse. I had given up the shoulder purse for the heavy-handled straw behemoth that could accommodate my bags of chips and spherical, neon-shelled chocolate candies.

As I trundled down the walkway towards the plane, I had my usual misgivings about the size of the seats in Coach, and the aisles themselves. I was okay going down the First Class aisle, because there were fewer seats, and they weren't filled yet. Enviously, I gazed mutely at the large seat space given to First Class passengers. Oh well, maybe I'll sit next to a thin person, so there will be more room. I had requested an aisle seat back towards the rear of the plane. I didn't like it back that far, but if I had to go to the bathroom, I wouldn't jar as many people getting there. It's sad when you have to plan things like this in advance, instead of looking forward to the trip itself. In my life, it was the details that counted most, so I would get the least amount of humiliation.

Another place where fat girls aren't welcome is on the modern airplane, that has economized everything, including the seats. Only someone with recent liposuction on her ass could comfortably fit in those Coach seats. Even the aisles were affected. They had added more seats, so they cut down the aisle space. It was going to be a very long trip indeed.

As I made my way sideways down the aisle, I would catch the disdainful (and worried) glances of the other passengers, who were already in their assigned seats. I could hear what they were thinking.

"Jeez, I hope she doesn't have the aisle seat in my row. I won't even be able to get my tray down from the looks of her. How does anybody let themselves get that big? (or from the women passengers, 'How did she let herself go like that? I'd rather be dead....')".

I was in luck. My seat partners were already asleep. I lengthened the seatbelt as much as I could. It felt like I was being cut in half. At least the "unfasten seatbelts" sign would come on after we were in the air.

"Ladies and gentlemen, this is your captain speaking. There will be a slight delay until we can taxi out to our runway."

No, no, no! We aren't even in the taxi line? This trip is going to be a nightmare, I thought, as I unfastened my ill-fitting seatbelt.

With eyes like a hawk spotting her prey, the flight attendant (a size 1) rushed down the aisle to my seat. Now if they could only do that when they were serving meals.

"I'm sorry, madam. The 'fasten seatbelt' sign is still on." She glared at my unfastened belt.

What is going to hit us? We hadn't gotten close to the taxi lane. Maybe the swallows of Capistrano had veered from their flight pattern, so I had to put my seatbelt on, just in case they bombarded the plane with bird droppings. Gimme a break! I grumbled to myself, as I breathed in and pulled the ends of the belt together over my stomach.

When we were finally airborne, I undid the torture-devised seatbelt and turned on my monitor in front of me, to see what they had for pre-recorded television selections.

When I saw the first choice, I grimaced.

Just great. (I use sarcasm a lot when I'm thinking.)

They were showing repeats of "Sex in the City." Thins in high heels.

Nope.

Hopefully, I looked for the on-board movie.

Terrific. (sarcasm again; I was nothing if not witty)

Tom Hanks going anorectic on that island with that damn beach ball.

I don't think so.

I bought a pair of headphones and turned on the music. I began digging into my bag stuffed between my legs. Good thing ol' eagle eye didn't see that the bag wasn't stored under my seat.

Fat chance. I would kick it further under the seat after I retrieved my goodies. They must hire stick flight attendants who hate fat people, so they look for ways to abuse them whenever they get the opportunity. I had experienced their "tender loving care" before.

"May I have two blankets, please?"

"You're only allowed one." This was said with undisguised contempt. Obviously, this human water buffalo couldn't cover that massive skin surface with one regular-sized blanket.

"I can see some extras up in that bin there."

"Those are for the First Class passengers."

"But this is Coach. Don't they have their own blankets?" (probably fur-lined)

"Do I need to get the Captain?"

"No, no, that's okay. Maybe I could get a soda?"

"We only have halves left for drinks. I'm sure you don't want a (calorie-laden) drink, do you?"

She would move grandly down the aisle after this last riposte, leaving me cold and dehydrated in my less-than-comfortable seat. My fellow travelers stared at the quivering masses of fat when I shivered uncontrollably under my napkin-sized airplane blanket. The other passengers were less than sympathetic. They made comments out loud, too.

"Good God Almighty. That is the fattest female I've ever seen."

"God forbid, the plane goes down, and we have to get past her to the exits."

"Remind me to read my magazine when the food is served. I don't want to watch her eat *before* my meal comes. It'll throw me right off my feed."

Ah, the joys of living among the thins, even in the air.

While on the plane this time, I needed to get into my stash before they served meals. All that waiting and worrying made me hungry. Of course, it didn't take much to get my appetite going. A photo of food could do it, and those airplane magazines are full of fine cuisine for rich folks staying at five-star hotels.

I knew I had made a mistake as soon as I took the proffered plastic glass of diet soda. The chocolate peanut-butter pieces had stuck to the inside of my mouth. I should have stocked up on the chocolate mints instead. I wouldn't need any liquid to keep the flow of food going down my gullet with those. Too late now. I could barely open my mouth to say "thank you" when the flight attendant handed me the cup of soda, and left the can on my foldout tray.

Damn. I had to go to the bathroom.

Fat girls make sure they go *before* they board the airplane. They know the plane bathrooms are off limits for them. The hellish cubicles are built for dwarves.

I waited until no one was in the aisle, and prayed the drink cart wasn't in the way. I also think there's a conspiracy among flight attendants to keep people in their seats, and out of their lacquer-coiffed hair. Their steel-fortress food and beverage carts take up the entire aisle. Passengers are trapped. If you do have the temerity to get out of your seat and you block their cart, you get the "evil eye" from them, and some choice words loudly enunciated in an irritated voice.

"Sorry, I need to go to the bathroom." You say this as softly as possible.

"You cannot GO TO THE BATHROOM right now." An echo in the Grand Canyon is less deafening.

So in addition to needing to pee, you are embarrassed by having it yelled to the world. Meekly you sit back down, cross your legs, and think of anything but waterfalls for the time it takes for the hellishly slow cart to pass. Mentally castigating the snotty attitudes of the Barbie-doll or Ken-doll flight attendants, you wish you were rich enough to fly First Class so you'd get decent treatment and big toilets.

It was going to be a battle between kidney damage and the airplane cubicle. Of course, I had to actually *get* there first. As I gazed up into the unsympathetic, cold eyes of the flight attendants handing out drinks, I knew I'd have to "gird my loins." Or in this case, acknowledge I was going to urinate in my seat if I didn't fight for the right to use the bathroom. Some fat girls will put on "old-people sanitary napkins" before they board, so they can pee in them during the flight rather than chance a trip to the lavatory.

The server thins in their form-fitting pantsuits made me so nervous I forgot to put up my lap tray before I tried to stand up. My stomach hit it. My drink and half-filled soda can flew into the air, splattering me and the closest thing to me – the flight attendant.

Disgustedly regarding the damage to her perfectly creased uniform, she exchanged a glance of "so-what-can-you-expect-from-a-fat-girl" irritation with the gay guy at the other end of the cart. Sopping delicately with a small napkin, she patted the wet spots. I wasn't offered anything to clean my area or me.

"I just had this pressed, and I have to do a turn-around back to L.A." She was talking to the other attendant, but she was looking at me hard.

The other bobble head nodded empathetically, while he smiled toothily at a good-looking guy in tight jeans sitting across from me .

With a look of utter contempt, the bimbo moved the cart a few feet ahead of herself in the aisle. I didn't dare look at her, as I silently pushed myself up completely by putting a hand on the seat in front of me. Guess it wasn't a gentle push.

"Hey, I'm trying to eat here," bellowed the man in front of me while he purposely leaned as far back as he could in his seat. My using his seat for support had pushed his still-uneaten lunch tray on his foldout table forward, so some of his dessert dripped over into his salad.

I mumbled an apology as I turned sideways to head down the aisle towards the potty.

As I passed, he muttered, "Fat cow. They should have put her in cargo." His seat companions suppressed grins.

I moved as quickly as I could towards the back of the plane. There were four toilets. Three of them had the OCCUPIED tab pulled across. I opened the door of the fourth, and winced when I saw the size of the room – definitely made for elves.

Oh, crap.

The doors of the other cubicles were starting to open. I'd be caught like a fat fish in a human net if the people came out of the doors at the same time. There wasn't room to maneuver. They'd have to make like church wafers to get by me. I had to get into that miniscule bathroom now.

With a heave, I threw my weight into the room. I reached behind me and locked the door. I was wedged between the sink and the toilet. If I could turn around I could be near enough to the toilet, so I could perch above it and go. There was no way I'd be able to actually reach the seat. In fact, at this point, I wasn't sure I could get out, much less go to the bathroom.

I grabbed the slender sink faucet and pulled myself forward a little. I just hoped it wasn't as fragile as it looked. The faucet came off in my hand.

Damn.

The paper towels were too far away to reach to stop the water spouting from the hole. Soon, water would leak underneath the door, and out into the corridor. It did - faster than I expected.

The flight attendants were called to the bathrooms. One of the passengers had noticed the seeping water, and punched the "Call" button to summon the flight attendant. I could hear everything through the door. I just couldn't move to back my way out through it.

When the flight attendant arrived and leaned over his seat, he pointed to the water.

"I think something broke in one of the restrooms."

The flight attendant knocked.

"Is everything all right in there? There's water coming from underneath the door. Did you forget to shut off the sink?"

I was desperately trying to plug the hole with whatever I could get my hands on. The only thing I could touch if I stretched out my arm was the mounted toilet-seat-cover apparatus. The seat-cover papers were flimsy at best. They were certainly not designed to soak up the amount of water gushing from the mutilated sink. But they would have to do.

The knocking on the door got more pronounced.

"Do you need any help? Can you open the door?"

Instead of answering, I watched the mini-flood soak the carpet, and look for the one place it could get away. It flowed pretty heavily under the door now. I could imagine the expressions on the faces of the flight attendants as it rushed over their shoes.

I could hear them talking.

"Go get the keys from the pantry."

One of them walked swiftly towards the back pantry. By this time, the passengers seated near the bathrooms became aware something was wrong. For one thing, the carpet under their feet was wet and squishy. Those who had removed their shoes were especially unhappy.

"Everything's just fine, folks. Had a little accident in one of the restrooms. We're going in to take care of the problem."

I was praying to whatever gods were listening. Maybe pagan gods were more accessible than the Christian God.

Please don't let them come in. I'll promise you anything. I'll never fly again. I'll...

In the middle of my fervent prayers, I felt the push of the door when it met my backside.

"Madam, can you move forward a little?"

If I could move, I wouldn't be in this situation, now would I?

Of course, I didn't say this out loud. I wouldn't want them to get angry.

"I'm so sorry. I think I'm stuck."

They were murmuring in low voices now.

"Tell the Flight Engineer we need to have the water shut off."

"But we might not be able to get it back on. We still have six hours of flight time. No one will be able to use the bathrooms."

"There's nothing we can do about that now. We've got to take care of this before it gets worse."

"Okay. On my way."

I could hear one of them moving away.

Oh God, this was my worst nightmare.

Not only was I trapped in a tiny plane toilet with water up to my ankles, I'd just taken away the toilets for over 200 people for the next six hours.

"Ma'am, we're turning off the water. Do you think you can move away from the door at all?"

I grunted and grabbed the paper-towel holder in front me. I pulled. It came off the wall.

I want to die right now. Don't wait, God, just kill me!

Since the pagan deities seemed unresponsive, I returned to my own.

The pushing on the door became harder. Maybe they'd gotten some burly men to help.

It started to move in. I was slowly being propelled towards the hole on the wall where the paper-towel holder used to be.

With a final massive push from them, I found myself away from the door, with my face pressed into the wall in front of me.

I tried to look over my shoulder.

I saw ol' eagle eye slip through the door.

Oh no, not her. She hates me already.

"I'm going to need some help in here. I won't be able to get her out by myself."

She announced this information in a voice that carried to the front of the plane.

"Does anyone have a rope, or something I can put around her? If we all pull, maybe we can pop her out."

Oh my God. Oh my God. I'll never live this down. I bet there is someone with a camera phone sending this whole thing to YouTube right this moment.

Someone passed in a huge belt strap designed to secure a humongous suitcase.

"Okay, now can you grab this and buckle it around your waist?"

A voice from outside yelled:

"Is it big enough to go around her?"

"Yes, I think so."

I reached behind me and took the wide belt from the skinny hands of the flight attendant, who would probably have nightmares about this the rest of her thin life. Or, she'd tell the story at Flight Attendant School. It would be part of their curriculum. A chapter entitled, "What to Do if a Fat Girl Gets Stuck in the Lavatory." There'd be pictures, of course.

I notched the belt in the last hole.

I whispered, "It's buckled."

The flight attendant hollered to the increasingly larger crowd outside.

"Now pass me the other one so I can attach it."

I felt the belt looped around the one at my waist in the back.

"I'm coming out. Be ready to pull."

This was so humiliating I could hardly stand it. They were going to play tug-of-war with me. Just then, the slack in the looped belt straightened out. I felt myself being hauled backwards.

"Everyone should stay back."

I didn't know whether she said that to clear the space in front of the bathrooms, or she was afraid I'd explode out like a fat missile and take out a few of the passengers.

I felt a sudden powerful jerk, and I was pulled outside the door. Everyone scattered. Even the guys who had pulled. When they saw me coming, they had dropped the belt and scooted back up the aisle.

When the belt was dropped so abruptly, I sat down in the water-soaked carpet outside the door.

At least I was outside the door, and not jammed in the entrance. That thought had crossed my mind. I'd look like a gigantic cork in a mammoth bottle.

"Okay folks, it's over. Go back to your seats."

Damn, the cell phone guy was still sending everything.

I tried to stand, but I was sliding around in the water. No one offered a hand. I finally got a grip on the door handle across from me, and pulled myself up.

The flight attendants led me back to my seat. It was the longest walk of my life.

My butt was wet, but I sat down as soon as I got there. I could feel the water leaching into the seat. It was another six hours until we landed, and I looked like I had wet my pants. Well, I still had to pee.

It already looks like I did, so here goes.

I felt the warm urine seeping into my clothes. I sighed. It was the only "warm" moment I'd had so far. Those adult sanitary napkins really looked good about now. Wish I'd put one on. I finally pulled my oversized purse into my lap to cover the spreading wet spots.

The flight attendant didn't even tell me to put it under my seat. Evidently, that was the least of their worries.

I was so miserable I didn't eat from my stash. I put on my headphones and closed my eyes. I didn't want to see the glares of the other passengers, who had lost their restrooms.

I kept my eyes shut, until I heard the announcement we were landing.

I waited until most of the passengers had left the plane. Most of them were up out of their seats, and standing in line to get off, as soon as they heard the announcement. I think the flight attendants knew there'd be hell to pay, if these toilet-deprived passengers weren't allowed off the plane as soon as it had stopped. They didn't even try to get them to sit back down while the plane was taxiing to its bay. These people were on a mission to get to the nearest bathroom. It wouldn't be a good idea to get in their way.

Evidently, the pilot had called ahead to let the airport know about the situation. As soon as the plane rolled to a stop, there was a ramp there. My fellow passengers just about ran out of that plane.

Needless to say, I waited until all of them had left, before I hauled myself up. My soaked clothes had plastered themselves to my ass. The flight attendants were coming down the aisle towards me, so I couldn't reach back and pull them away from my legs and buttocks.

Wonderful. One final embarrassing moment.

As I made my way sideways down the aisle towards the exit, the flight attendants backed into the rows of empty seats so I could get by. It was the quietest that plane had ever been. Nobody said a word. I just hoped my wet clothes weren't too stuck in my ass. That was the last view they'd have of me.

I kept my eyes on the carpet while I headed for the exit.

By the time I reached the entrance to the airport, the other passengers were gone. They were probably calling their doctors or lawyers.

Nothing worse could possibly happen to me on this trip, I thought, as I spotted my parents waiting alone at the boarding gate.

"What happened to you? You look as big as the plane. Did you just get off it, or did it get off you?"

Trust my father to say exactly the wrong thing

Chapter 9

Home – Part 3

When we got to the house, I lugged my bags to my room. Everything looked the same. No comfort food, though. I had removed it all before I left for college. It definitely wasn't good to be home.

I hadn't eaten for the last six hours. I certainly couldn't eat any of the remaining meals on the flight. Not with what had happened. I was famished.

I put on one of my muumuus, and walked downstairs to the kitchen. Mother looked at me.

"Well, we'll need to go shopping, won't we?"

She meant *I* would have to go shopping.

I wanted to put it off as long as possible, because I remembered what it was like to shop as a fat girl. I had promised myself I would never again be sent to the fat-clothes section in a store

I had those awful nightmares, when you wake up dripped in sweat and curled in a ball on your bed. My memories came from all the times I was treated like a fat person, a second-class citizen. Especially when I had to buy clothes.

I would reluctantly go shopping as a last resort. I hadn't been to the **Misses** section since I was twelve, and starting to pack on the pounds.

Mother would head directly for the **Women's** stacks and racks. She would start at the **L** or **XL** tags on the clothes racks. I'd stand there like a dumb beast, while she put them up against me. She'd gesture towards the dressing rooms, while she kept looking. I would take some she had selected, and make my way there, trying not to knock things off the tables as I went by. She would come in and start with the **Large** sizes first. I prayed I could get the pants up my legs. Most of the time, we'd have to go to the **Extra Large** items. It would take an hour to find one outfit.

I think Mother gave up on me, after she had gotten me in a girdle. After that, she would drop me off at the mall, give me money, and tell me what time she would pick me up.

I would try to find stores that had big mannequins in the windows. I'd look for size 22 or 24 on the sales tags. No point in going in the expensive ones. Their sizes didn't go up that high. I had found it totally humiliating, when I tried to find things in some of the smaller boutiques. They had all the cute cool clothes the thins at school wore. The sales ladies were part of my nightmare.

If I didn't get any size that fit when I was in the dressing room, I never let the saleswoman get me more sizes. She would wait outside the door. I would step back, so she couldn't see my ankles.

"Do you need any help? Can I get you anything else to try on?"

Yeah. Is there a rack for girls that doesn't say the word 'Oversized' in orange paint, on a 14" by 16" placard clamped about it, but has great slim-looking clothes for fat girls, that make you look two sizes smaller?

Of course, I didn't say that. Why rub it in? I had the damn dressing-room mirror in front of me, anyway. If I were really lucky, I'd get the dressing room with the three-sided mirror. Even if I tried to see myself quickly, I'd still briefly have to look at my flabby thighs and butt. They were like giant loaves of yeast, rolling against each other.

Maybe they had a film for girls like me. "Cellulite Gone Wild!" I guessed it wouldn't be as popular as those party videos, with those "God's-gift-to-men" thins pulling up their shirts, or pushing their small asses into the camera for all they were worth. Maybe the Internet perverts that love obese girls would buy it.

Why don't they have oversized salespeople in stores? It's even worse to have these small Asian women wait on girls like me. They think American girls are decadently fat, anyway.

"Can I help you find something?"

I hadn't spotted her behind the rack of new spring dresses. Ordinarily, I get as far away as possible from them.

"No, thanks, I'm just looking." (for anything that doesn't make me look like the Hindenburg Blimp)

Crap.

Sometimes you'd get the insistent ones.

"What size are you looking for?" She'd be trying to see all of me in one glance. It wouldn't work. She walked around me, like she was touring a cruise ship.

"That's okay. I think I'll just look around." Leave me alone, you never-have-to-worry-about-weight, can-eat-anything-but-doesn't-gain-weight woman!

"Okay, then, but if you need me, I'll be over there." She would give me a last glance, and move on to skinny people, who probably had more money and could buy more stuff, anyway.

One horrible time, I was trying to find the largest size of jeans in a stack on a table in the middle of the Women's section. Half a manikin was sitting atop one of the stacks.

I got excited when I thought I saw a size 22 on the bottom of her pile. I pulled too hard. The manikin's head left its body and rolled underneath one of the racks. I caught the rest of her in one hand while holding the pile of jeans on the table with the other. A customer passing by with her young daughter remarked to the frightened child when the head dropped off the manikin's body. "It's alright, honey. It's not a real person."

My face beet red, I pushed the manikin's body upright on top of the jeans' pile. I looked around desperately for the lost head, but didn't see it. By this time, a saleswoman was making her irritated way in my direction.

She glared at me.

"I'll take care of this. Perhaps the Larger Woman area is more appropriate for you."

I kept my head down, like a linebacker making for the other team after the quarterback's call on the field. In my case, I was trying to exit the store before a crowd gathered. Not one of my fondest memories.

Anyway, on these clothes-hunting trips, after a frustrating hour pulling on clothes that wouldn't fit, I would maybe find two things that *might* fit, if I wore my long sweater over them. It wasn't over yet, though. I had one last embarrassing stop to make.

God, it was humiliating to see the slim saleswomen's eyes when they rang up my items.

My two shirts would look like a tower of cloth, compared to what the skinny thing behind me was buying. She would have four wispy tops with shoestring ties to hold them up. You could barely see them, when she placed them on the counter next to mine.

One time behind me in the line to pay, I had this smug stick-thin woman with her tiny jeans slung casually over her arm. She hollered to her husband, "Make sure they're a size zero, or they'll be too big."

I finally gave up on the mall stores. Mother began dropping me off at the big box store with the food franchise. You know the rest of the story.

Lying to Myself

Now, I was older, but not a bit wiser. I had succumbed to the fat-girl denial, with all its permutations. I had let the fat cells back in. They had lain dormant for two years. I had allowed them to be reactivated, with my disastrous eating habits in Hawaii. Checking my wrist to see if I was putting on weight each day, became once a week, then once a month, whenever I thought about it, and finally, not at all. My OCD worked beautifully for my delusional state of mind. I forgot what reality is, not what I wanted it to be.

Just an observation here to the skinny folks turning the back of this book over, to see a picture of the author. There are fat people around you who want to take a quick peek at the actual contents, as soon as you leave the area. I know. You didn't notice them. As usual, so as not to be too obvious, the fat person will wait until the thin one (you just know that's you) moves away from the rack, before picking this off the shelf. If a fat girl chooses to buy this or any other item in the bookstore, there's that fun trip to the counter. There's nothing more humorous for the slim jim at the register, than a fat girl going to the counter with a book with "fat" in the title. The fat girl always hopes to get the one token overweight woman, to ring up her purchases. At least, she'd think the fat girl was buying another diet book, just like *she* did all the time with her employee discount. But no, it's the guy who's still the same cadaverous weight he was in high school, who's waiting.

In my bingeing in Hawaii, I had forgotten the truisms that ruled my life, and the lives of any other fat girls.

"You look really good. Have you lost weight?" were the only words that could fill me up. They were like a seven-course meal. Better even. They are what I lived to hear. Fat girls are really depressed most of the time, because they never hear that golden rhetorical question. Fat girls are not jolly receptacles of mirth. They are ambulatory open wounds.

Fat girls get in the way, in a society that dotes on thinness. Men noticed me, when I was in my dark slim jeans. I didn't have to buy fat shirts to cover my thighs. I had to order over the Internet for sizes lower than 2. Happiness was a size 2; ecstasy was a size 1. Paradise was a size 0.

This is the great truth for girls. You don't have to go to a guru to get this message. Ask any girl; ask her mother; ask any rich man. If they're honest (mothers and other girls are spitefully so), they'll lay it out for you. Nobody likes fat chicks, not even other fat chicks.

I thought being thin was the only way to survive. You want to die skinny. Even if they're going to cremate you and load you in a furnace, they might lay you out for people to see first. I can hear my mother now, "If only she'd lost some weight, her life would have been so different." You are pitied or disliked by everybody, if they're thinking about you at all. Absolutely nobody likes a fat person, unless they're standing next to one to look good.

I carried typed celebrity quotes in my wallet. When I'd feel the urge to eat, I'd get them out, and read each one ten times. If I were alone, I'd say them out loud. The Duchess of Windsor had it right, "You can never be rich enough or too thin enough." She got a king. Balanchine said, "I want to see bone," when he saw his female dancers perform. Female ballet dancers revered him. They didn't buy into the desperate fat-girl truism, that girls' bodies should be "whatever God gave you." Fat girls hear the mantras over and over again. *You are special; you are unique; you should love your body. God gave us just one body for this life.* I concluded God must have looking the other way, when fat girls were created.

In my dreams, I wanted to be the Duchess of Windsor. Balanchine would have loved to look at me. I was a fat girl crying out for affection. I needed to be thin, so I could be loved. Even admired. Everyone told me so.

I wanted to count my ribs through my clothes, with just the slightest touch of my fingertips. I yearned to lie on my back and feel my hipbones, like knives that can cut paper. Fat calipers not being able to measure any fat on me, could calibrate my happiness. My contentment equaled the amount of space between my thighs.

The thin world wants you to believe even God doesn't love fat girls. God forbid, you end up a fat girl. You will have no life. From personal experience, I have found the great religious truth about God. I know God must absolutely be a man. Fat girls get it. It's a huge cosmic joke on girls. Boys rule the world. Males wrote all the holy books. Remember that Adam and Eve story? Eve never had a chance. Everything was going to be blamed on her, no matter what. She took one of his ribs, for God's sake. How low can you go! It's all her fault in every religion.

From what I saw in high school, boys didn't pay attention to most girls, except to have sex with them. But only with those thin girls with cheerleader bodies. They definitely didn't want fat girls, even for sex, unless they were all that was available. Fat girls were easy for them to use and then throw away, like a dirty Kleenex. Girls who are fat are desperate for love. They're good for first-time sex for boys. Fat slobs are forgettable practice for the real thing – a hot girl.

I thought I had won the dating lottery, when the school's quarterback stopped me in the hall one day in high school.

"Hey, how's it goin'?"

So okay, I ignored the grammatical errors. He looked so good in that tight polo shirt, his biceps straining the thin cloth, until I thought it would tear apart while I was looking at it. And his cargo shorts were low on his slender hips. I could see his boxers. They were red. I fell in love with the color red, at that exact moment.

Good God in heaven, he is such a stud, I thought, as I casually looked him up and down, like a new territory I was going to survey. I had just left World Geography, so I guess big unknown land masses were the first thing to come to mind.

Boy, I'm glad it hadn't been Biology, I chuckled to myself, as zygotes and long-tailed, wild swimming sperm impregnated my cerebellum.

Impregnated? Oh, I am a bad, bad girl. I had to make like I was rearranging the books in my arms, to keep from laughing out loud.

"Say, could you meet me after school by my car? I have somethin' I wanna ask you. Do you know which car is mine?"

Who didn't know the quarterback's car, I almost sighed, as I said, "Yes, it's the yellow Corvette with the black stripes down the hood, isn't it?"

Jeez, did I have to be so descriptive? He must think I watch him arrive and leave in his cool car! He always had a load of girls gossiping among each other, while they were waiting for him to roll into the school parking lot in the morning, and a bunch of airheads waving goodbye, when he gunned that big engine and roared away in the afternoon. I had casually walked by the parking lot a couple of hundred times when I knew he would be there. I figured I could look, anyway, even if I never got a chance to do anything else.

Well, it was me he was asking to meet him today. So there, all you fake-tan cheerleaders!

Inwardly, I gloated, as he nodded and moved away to join his football buddies, beckoning to him down the hall.

Now I knew what they meant about walking on air, I chortled to myself, closing my locker and almost skipping above ground to my Advanced Calculus class.

The hours went by like a turtle with arthritis. When the final bell rang, I got to my locker, threw my books in, and rushed to the Girls' bathroom close by. First, I quickly checked under each stall, except the Handicapped one since I was probably the only one who used it, to make sure I was alone. Next, I spread several rough brown paper towels on top of each other in three layers. I thought stacking them would be the best way. If I laid them out side by side, the edges wouldn't be even. The school must buy the cheapest paper towels and toilet paper they could find.

Maybe they thought if they purchased the scratchy kind, we girls would use less of it.

I took out the small make-up compact, with the dark shade of pancake powder and the tortoise shell cover. I had sacrificed one hamburger combo to have the money to buy this particular compact. I liked the feel of the cover, when I ran my finger over it in the Cosmetics aisle. It looked like an actual shell you'd find on a beach.

Then came the lipstick tube, filled with the reddest shade I could find, No. 532 on the color chart, ***Fire Engine Red***. That cost me an extra bag of fries and an apple pie. But it was worth it. Its shape resembled the perfect girl's figure, with its tiny gold waist and silver top and bottom. It was placed carefully on the towels on the counter next to the sink.

Next, I lifted out my large comb with the extra teeth. The humidity made my hair tough to handle. If I didn't plaster the strongest-hold hair gel on it each morning, it would rise up like Medusa's writhing-snakes hair all over my head. I set the comb down next to the larger compact. My OCD grabbed my hand, and made it put the trio in descending order of size on the paper towels I had laid out.

I felt like an Indian putting on war paint before battle, as I patted the powder all over my face, and ran the lipstick over my lips several times. I ran water over the comb, before I pulled it through the heavy mass as hard as I could. I tucked any stray runaway curls behind each ear.

Since I usually avoid mirrors like the plague, I hadn't opened my eyes through the whole process. When I had finished with my hair, I slowly opened them.

You don't look half bad, I thought with an anticipatory shiver, as I loaded my cosmetic arsenal back in my purse in the order in which I had taken them out.

I stepped back from the mirror to see how I looked from a distance.

Pretty damn good. My mouth opened wide in a white-toothed grin outlined in red.

As I stopped to take one more look at my glorious self before wowing the waiting quarterback, I heard voices outside the swinging green bathroom doors.

Crap, just my luck. I had forgotten about the cheerleaders who stayed after school to practice their silly little routines that threw their butts around to show school spirit. A gaggle of them were starting to come through the door. I ran for the Handicapped stall, and bolted it behind me just in time.

They better make this quick, or I won't get out of here in time to meet my Corvette Prince Charming in the parking lot. I glowered at the green metal door in front of me.

They were chattering in those high voices, that only petite blondes with tight sweaters have.

I tuned them out, when they started cattily dispensing with any other human beings who were less perfect than they were. That took in most of the school.

I groaned. *I'll never get out of here!*

Well, I might as well relax. I sat on the closed lid of the extra-wide toilet, and rummaged through my purse to find something to read. I always read wherever I went. I couldn't believe people actually didn't read all the time. Each summer, I would pick a Nobel Prize-winning author and read everything that he or she had written. More "hes" then "shes." Even the Nobel Prize Committee was sexist. One time I had to ask Mother to drive me across town to the only library that had Hemingway's **A Moveable Feast.** It was the only book I couldn't find in the local library.

"Why do we have to go ten miles to get one book?"

"I've read everything he wrote, except that one. Our library doesn't have it."

I had the forlorn hope that she would compliment me on reading every book Hemingway had written, including all his short stories in anthologies.

"Why don't you read something else? My friend Irma at work gave me the newest romance novel. I'll let you borrow it. Just make sure you don't get anything on it."

Not if my life depended on it, I thought.

Romance novels are for those who anticipate having romance in their lives. I didn't see that happening in the near future.

I'd bring a book to the breakfast or dinner table to read. Since I wasn't included in any conversations going on, my parents and sister ignored my habit of propping a hardback in front of me while I ate. It also kept them from pointing out all my flaws, since the book was covering my face. I could eat in peace and satisfy my OCD reading ritual at the same tine.

When I had been in a rush one morning, I had left my breakfast book on my little table next to my bed. I almost had a panic attack.

"Mother, I need to go get my book."

"Sit down without it. Your breakfast will get cold."

Since my breakfast, like all my meals, was diet-driven and unappetizing, I didn't see how it made any different whether the mush was hot or not.

"I'll be just a minute."

"You read too much, anyway. Boys don't like girls who are smarter than them."

Okay, then. That must be the reason I've been dateless for my whole high school career. And why would I want some guy who was dumber than paint anyway?

As usual, all these retorts were thoughts, not actual out-loud words spoken back to Mother. She'd want to pick a fight. My sister was already snickering.

I was beginning to fidget in my chair. Mother regarded me balefully.

"My goodness, if it's going to get you eating and on your way, go ahead and get your book."

She turned her attention back to my social butterfly sister.

"Honey, what do you have planned for today?"

The unspoken innuendo was that I had nothing going for me today, or any other day, while my sibling had gossip about boys and their attributes that made my mother chuckle with glee.

When I returned to the kitchen table, my food was gone. I looked in the sink and there it was, floating mush. Mother had run water in it.

I didn't bother asking her. It was obvious that she had forgotten she had given me permission to get my book to read at the kitchen table, while I spooned diet cereal into my mouth. Nobody had reminded her, either. My father seldom spoke, and my sister wasn't interested in what I was doing, unless it was something she could maliciously share with her tribe of Barbie wannabes.

I sighed audibly, but I was the only one to hear it. Mother had already left for work, as had my father. My sister had been picked up by one of her giggle crew, since they were all too good to ride the school bus or walk to school.

I scrubbed out my cereal bowl in the sink, got my book bag from my room, checked to see that Mother had put in my lunch money in the zippered sandwich baggie in the front pocket of the bag, and shambled off to another place where I was ignored and belittled.

But today was different. As soon as the blonde bubbleheads left the restroom, I'd make my appearance, with my new face, in the parking lot, where the number one boy in high school was waiting just for me.

I couldn't find anything to read in my purse, so I looked at the writing carved into the back of the toilet door. I must admit I didn't expect to see anything in this stall, since it was for handicapped students. I mean, what would they write, even if their dysfunctional brains and bodies allowed them to.

For a "wheelchair good time," call …

But actually, someone had written something in permanent marker. I bent closer to see.

"I may be not so smart, but at least I'm not fat like…." I didn't need to read anymore, to know that my name was at the end of that scrawl.

"Crap, even the SPED kids thought they were better than me," I said, under my breath, as I tried to smear the writing with some spit on a piece of toilet paper.

Just as I realized the Nazi toilet paper was good for something, as it had just rubbed through my name with its rough texture, I heard the girls outside the stall mention my name.

I sat back with satisfaction. They must have heard about my rendezvous after school. Nothing went past these idiots when it came to gossip.

"Hey, did you hear about Rob meeting that fat slob after school today? I bet she thinks it's some kind of date."

Well, I wouldn't go that far, but I was hopeful, I thought, as I waited for the next comment. Surely, it would be about how envious they were, how jealous, how absolutely angry they were that I was seeing the best boy on campus in a couple of minutes.

If they get their skinny little asses out of here, I fumed, while sticking the used "toilet-paper eraser" in the tampon container (without looking, of course).

"Do you actually think she would get the idea Rob was going to ask her out?"

Their laughter echoed off the green tile on the walls.

"Nobody's that stupid. He only dates us."

"I doubt she's had a single date since she waddled onto campus."

Another round of high-pitched guffaws bounced off the bathroom walls.

"He told one of the players he was going to ask her to do his homework for him. He said she'd be so grateful he was talking to her, that she'd do it all year."

"What class is he failing this time?"

"Some dummy math class he needs to graduate."

"Well, nobody screws him for his brains!"

At this last remark, they just about rolled on the floor, doubled up with laughter, except they wouldn't think of touching such a disgusting surface.

They changed the subject to what each was wearing to the prom, and how low-cut their dresses could be, without the old bitches who were prom chaperones, finding out.

Without realizing it, I was quietly crying, the tears making wet funnels down through the make-up, to the edge of the lipstick on my quivering lips. I probably looked like that mass murderer clown, who probably had accumulated more friends than I did.

I used my sleeve to wipe my face, like a two-year-old. I was probably acting like a pre-teen. The entire scenario seemed like a script out of one of those awful teen movies "Rich handsome quarterback asks ugly fat girl to meet him. She thinks he wants to ask her out, since he must know she is the real thing, not like those superficial, pretty, stupid girls he usually spent his time with. Unloved fat girl overhears the popular girls discussing the obvious fact that he was using her, and would never ever think of spending any quality time with such a nondescript nonentity, even if she was smart. He intended to be nice to her, until he got his assignments from her. What else was she good for? His reputation was at stake, for one thing. It was bad enough setting up an after-school thing, so he could set the trap. It's a good idea his buddies told the girls what he was up to. It would be gruesome if they thought he was seriously considering doing anything, or going anywhere with the cipher on campus."

Yep. I had seen that movie several times. I always hoped the boy would realize what a true blue girl the smart one was. That he would see under the surface what a fine person she was, and how artificial the blonde bobble heads were.

Nope. Didn't end like that, unless the ugly duckling was really a swan underneath. I had no swan persona.

After the gossip girls left, I went to the sink and washed the makeup off. I left the school campus by the back entrance.

When I got home, I went to my room, laid down, hugged my pillow, and pulled the covers over my head.

I must have fallen asleep, because the next thing I heard was Mother calling us down to breakfast. Hiding my face as usual behind my book, I wasn't in the mood to read. I went through a couple of scenarios for my eventual eye contact with Rob.

He would be visibly upset, in a nice way.

"Hey, I waited for you for over an hour. I thought we'd maybe catch a movie this weekend. What happened?" He would peer anxiously into my lovely, sparkling, blue eyes, as I gazed compassionately into his warm brown ones.

"One of the teachers caught me, and asked me to help her with a lab she was setting up for tomorrow." I was brilliant in science, too.

He would be instantly relieved that I hadn't stood him up, and we would make plans for Friday night.

Or, maybe it would go like this:

One of his groupie cheerleaders would tentatively approach me, as I was about to enter my Advanced Placement English class.

"Rob sent me over 'cause he thinks you might be mad at him for some reason. He was really disappointed when you didn't meet him after school. He wants to know if he did something wrong."

I would look impatient and super intelligent, as I deigned to respond before closing the classroom door, and leaving her standing alone in the hall.

"Have him check with me later."

In my dreams, these conversations would take place. The reality was a tad different. There was no dialogue at all. I saw Rob in the hall, and glanced his way with a hopeful expression. I thought he was going to come over to talk with me, as he headed in my direction. Maybe dreams really do come true for fat girls.

Not very likely. At least for this fat girl.

He walked right past me, and threw his arm around a sloped-shouldered girl behind me.

"Hey babe, could you meet me after school in the parking lot? I have somethin' I wanna ask you."

I guess he had a list of poor dateless girls who might be more than willing to do his homework for him. He probably hadn't even waited ten minutes for me, before he jumped into his expensive car and drove away.

He never bothered to speak to me the rest of the year. Miss Humpback must have come through for him, or some other female nonentity who would be thrilled to do anything he asked.

Although I was used to rejection from boys, I decided to remain philosophical about the whole experience. Of course, philosophy only went so far. In my darkest moments when I suffered humiliation from being fat, I would curse the gods, or be finally convinced that misogyny ruled the day for girls like me. Since no higher deity had intervened on those occasions when I was taunted and teased because of my weight, I determined that God must be a male. He has been laughing up his proverbial sleeve from the beginning. After all, no female deity would make women fat. She'd know the hell on earth they would face.

Being thin wins it all – tiny clothes, good-looking guys, envious friends, and parents who don't have a clue. They're just happy to show you off to their critics, who made innuendoes about fat camps, unhealthy home eating, and irresponsible parenting. Why wouldn't a fat girl starve or throw up? Some fat girls did both. They even created a name for them – bulimianorectic. If bulimia hadn't worked so well and so fast for me, I might have given that combo a try.

High school traumatic memories aside, as it was, though, this current post-Hawaii part of my life was drastically barren. I was home again with my parents. And I was a fat girl once more. I had maxed out my credit card for the ticket back to the mainland. There was no hidden junk food in my room. Mother had sold my car when I left for Hawaii. I didn't have a job. The summer lay before me, like a stretch of endless dismal days.

I needed a plan. Otherwise, my depression would lock me in this room. My anxiety would keep me from functioning. I still had my health insurance until September. Maybe I could get Phentermine legally from a local doctor. I hadn't seen our family doctor in years. With my fat and thin cycles, he might detect something. My fluctuating weight and altered appearance would make him suspicious. I didn't want him to know what I had become.

I opened my laptop, and looked for general practitioners in the area. I would ask for help to lose the 60 pounds I had gained over the last two years. I would convince them the weight gain was causing my depression and anxiety. My emotional eating was the cause of my condition. I just need something to help me control my eating. That should be enough to get a prescription for Phentermine. I knew it was prescribed for morbid obesity. Unfortunately, I was sure I qualified.

I considered going back to the diet clinics. But I couldn't face the girls, who were waiting for their drug to drop their weight to skeletal dimensions. It would be too humiliating. Fat girls didn't go to diet dens until they were skinny. I knew the rules. I would be unwelcome – a grotesquerie among the diet elite.

I thought I'd have more luck with a male doctor than a female. A female might catch on. A male might be susceptible to the con. They are sure they know the dysfunctional emotional state girls get into. They usually don't have a clue. Emotions are still a mysterious aspect of female physiology, for male doctors in particular.

Mother had let me use her car, after I dropped her off at work. I had to promise her I would park a block away to pick her up.

"Now, I get off at 5, so be here a little early, so you can park one block over."

"I can pull up right in front, so you don't have to walk."

She looked at pitilessly.

"You can barely fit under the steering wheel with the seat back as far as it will go. Do you think I want my friends to see you picking me up?"

Another rhetorical question. I made like I had something in my eye, as I reached for the Kleenex in my purse. Mother had already exited the car, and was up the block towards the entrance of the company she worked for. She never looked back.

I had made an appointment with a general practice physician about five miles from our house. I was told to come early, to fill out paperwork. But Mother had me drive her to work an hour ahead of my appointment time, so I had quite a bit of time to kill before my appointment. After spending time with Mother in the car, I felt an emotional binge eating fit come on.

I spotted a donut shop on my way to the doctor's office. When I stopped in their parking lot, I hesitated for a moment.

Why should I let Mother treat me like that? I should have just driven right up to her building.

As I got ready to scarf down a dozen donuts, I played the dialogue tape in my head about how the conversation would have gone, if I had ignored her direct orders about where to drop her off and pick her up.

"Mother, let me drop you off at the front of your building. It won't be such a long walk for you. I heard you telling Dad that your arthritis was kicking up."

She would glare at me after looking at how I was situated under the steering wheel. The seat belt wouldn't reach around my waist. It seemed to look accusingly at me, when I stuffed it between the front seats.

"You must be joking. What if someone sees you from work? I'd be so embarrassed. I told everyone you lived out-of-state. If they saw who was driving, the water cooler gossips would have a field day. No, you will do as I say. I can put up with the arthritis better than I could, trying to explain who you were. Those other secretaries all have slim daughters. I've seen the photos in frames on their desks."

Without her saying anything, I knew only my sister's picture decorated her desk in her cubicle. And I didn't want to hear her say it out loud.

I would listen to hear any kindness or compassion in her voice, as I struggled to lift the steering wheel away from my stomach.

"Mother, I'm sorry I've put on so much weight. I've been pretty stressed out lately. Do you have any idea how awful I feel when you're disappointed in me?"

She hadn't been listening at all. The car door was already closing.

So there I was, sitting dejectedly in the parking space the greatest distance from the door of the donut shop. Even though it wore me out to walk so far, I had already learned what people thought of a fat girl getting out of her car, in front of a place they assumed she wouldn't think of being. I couldn't use the drive-thru, because my arm wouldn't reach far enough to get the box of donuts. The underarm flab would sit on the shelf of the rolled-down window, like compacted mountains of sand on a wet beach. So, I knew I'd have to go in.

Last month, a new donut franchise had opened up near our home. It was too far to walk, so I had come home from school, and asked Mother if I could go to Wal-Mart to look at clothes.

"Good idea. Then you can see what you want, and you won't need me to go with you. Here are the keys to my car."

Without thinking, I had seen a parking spot close to the entrance and pulled in.

The empty spot next to me suddenly filled with a big family van, full of preteens and their harried parents.

I fought to get out sideways from under the steering wheel when I opened the car door. The kids in the van had been hollering about what they wanted in the store. As I concentrated on not bruising myself, as I tried to find the least fatty area to use to get from beneath the wheel, I hadn't paid attention to what was happening in the van.

As I grunted and pulled at myself to get out, the silence from the van caught my attention. Without looking, I assumed the squalling kids and their parents had gotten out before me, and were noisily choosing their dozen donuts, while chewing on the free ones everybody got standing in line to be waited on.

But that wasn't the case. The sliding door of the van was open, but the kids had not gotten out. The parents' doors were also open, but they had also remained inside.

While I was maneuvering across the seat on the final stage of extricating myself from Mother's car, I hastily glanced up at the crew next to me.

Bad idea. Their mouths were all agape, while their separate pairs of eyes looked like they were popping from their sockets. They looked like a school of goldfish, transfixed by the pieces of fish food dropped into their bowl.

Oh crap.

The kids started to comment, while the parents were trying now to get them out and into the shop as quickly as possible.

"Mom, what's she trying to do?"

The mother stepped in front of the door to block their view.

"Now come on, you'll be late for school if we don't get you out and get your donuts."

The preteens were not to be denied the sight of the gigantic human, wrestling with the steering wheel and the seat back. Their necks craned around the mother on both sides.

"Is she stuck?"

"That is the fattest lady I've ever seen."

The father had pulled each of them out, and was pushing them towards the shop door.

"Daddy, is she coming in, too?"

They looked aghast.

"If she eats donuts, she won't be able to get back in her car, will she?"

I could see the reddened neck of the embarrassed father, as he shoved the last of the four through the door.

I had lowered my eyes fast, when I discovered what was happening. I could hide my eyes, but I couldn't stop from hearing what they were saying. The words were like little knives being thrown at me. I started to cry, as I pulled myself back into the car. I left the donut parking lot as fast as I could. The tears were affecting my eyesight, so at the first gas station I saw, I drove in and stopped.

I chastised myself out loud, while hitting the steering wheel, as if it was the cause of the problem.

"For heaven's sake, you've heard worse. You could have just ignored them and gone in for your dozen donuts. What a coward you are! Now you're feeling like crap, and, worse, you don't have any binge food."

As I was drying my eyes, I glanced out of my car window, to see that I had stopped at a gas station with a food store attached. A slow smile crept across my tear-streaked face. It was almost like I had beaten them, after all.

Chapter 10

Fat Checkup

When I got to the doctor's office, I handed the receptionist my health card and co-pay. She made a copy of the card and gave it back to me. Then I was given a clipboard, that already had a sheath of official-looking papers attached. Unlike the ubiquitous pink form, these listed every disease known to man. It also asked if I had any history of heart problems, blood pressure. cholesterol, diabetes, mental problems and a whole page of others.

Whoa. Mental problems? How much space ya got.

By the time I was through completing the paperwork, and giving the clipboard back to the receptionist, my name was called. Perfect timing. I liked things to be perfect.

"Let's get your weight, shall we?"

I hadn't stepped on a scale in two years. Not since I didn't care what and how much I was eating. This was going to hurt.

I tried not to look at the bar as she moved it. But I could hear it, as it moved heavily from notch to notch – 100, 150. Then the smaller bar across the numbers. 155, 160, 165, 170. 180.

Damn, I hadn't realized how bad my weight had gotten. This is terrible.

It was stopping, thank goodness. The medical assistant recorded it in my chart. I didn't want to see her face. I was at least 45 pounds over what I was supposed to weigh.

"This way, please."

She put me in an examining room.

Please, please, don't ask me questions. I just want to see the doctor, tell him my fat-girl sob story, and get my amphetamine prescription.

As she was taking my blood pressure, the doctor came in. My blood pressure was a little high. I hoped it wasn't going to be a problem.

"What's going on?"

Here we go.

"Well, I'm 'way overweight, as you can see." I laughed nervously.

I tried to keep my hands from shaking. I felt like I was going to have a panic attack. I'd had several when I was a kid. I could feel perspiration forming on my forehead and upper lip. My heart was picking up speed.

Good thing she's not taking my blood pressure now.

I knew he wouldn't give me an amphetamine if I looked stressed.

Calm down, I told myself. *You can do this. Think of the goal. Keep focused on the plan.*

I brushed my hand across my face as I put my hair behind my ears.

Fortunately, he hadn't looked up from the chart.

"What do you think has contributed to the weight gain?"

About two years of dedicated eating.

I couldn't tell him I had an addiction. No possibility of uppers then.

"My appetite has seemed out of whack for about a year."

About 15 years to be exact.

Not a good thing for him to know.

"Anything unusual happen to cause a change?"

Did he have a couple of hours?

"Not really. I just seemed to have developed this ravenous appetite."

Let's see if I get lucky.

"I thought maybe there might be something I could take to curb it."

"Well, I'd like to do a full drug panel before I prescribe anything. I want to make sure there isn't something we could miss if I put you on medication."

Crap.

Not what I wanted to hear.

"Are you getting enough exercise? Do you belong to a gym?"

Yeah, right. I just love gyms.

Fat people on treadmills; fat people in the water; fat people doing aerobics.

I don't think so.

Fat girls don't like to see other fat girls, unless they're not as fat.

"I do a lot of walking."

"Okay then. I'll have my assistant give you a diet plan you can follow, and a form for the blood work. Make an appointment for two weeks from now. Your blood work should be back by then, and we can see how your diet is going."

He got up. I followed him to the front desk. A skinny assistant gave me a 1200-calorie diet sheet.

Hell, I eat that much in two minutes.

And why do they have a thin girl handing out the diet sheets? It's adding "insult to injury." These girls never had to follow an

205

awful diet plan in their skinny little lives. What do they know about our suffering? I was not in a good mood.

"Thanks"

I took the forms, walked out of the office, and threw them in the nearest trash can.

Now I was depressed, angry, and ready for a full-on panic attack. With no prescription for Phentermine.

I still had $80.00, after the $20 I had used for my co-pay.

Waste of money I could have used to buy my food fix. Where's the nearest store? I need some comfort food.

Arizona heats up to about oven temperature in May. It was 92 degrees by 10:00AM. I didn't care if it was a "dry heat." Fat girls don't do well in heat. The perspiration that had started in the doctor's office had become a veritable river, flowing from my head, across my face, and dripping like a damn multi-layered waterfall down the creases of my neck. My muumuu was sticking to me. As I walked to Mother's car, I unobtrusively tried to pull it away from my legs. The sweat running in rivulets down my arms wasn't helping the situation. I missed catching hold of the cloth in the back, because my hands were slick. I finally pulled enough away, so it didn't outline my haunches and legs, like meat ready to be hung up in a butcher's freezer.

I had red splotches on my arms, calves, and ankles. The sun was really doing a job on me. Since I couldn't walk without my fleshy thighs stuck together, the chafing from the heat was definitely starting to hurt. I couldn't get my hand between them to separate them, while I was wobbling towards the car. Besides, I might have been arrested for public indecency. This was turning into a crappy day, and it was still morning.

I got in the car, put the key in the ignition, and immediately pulled up my soaked muumuu to look at the damage between my thighs. I should have waited to do that.

I heard people talking as they moved past my car.

"What on earth is she doing?"

"Maybe she's looking for something she dropped."

"Between her legs?"

"Well, maybe she's sick. Should we go over to check?"

My head was still down between my legs.

No! No! No! Can't I get a break here? They'll think I'm even more disgusting if they see my dress up, my hands holding my mounds of thighs apart, and my head right in the middle.

Too late. I could hear knocking on the driver's side window.

"Is there something we can do?"

Go away! I thought frantically.

As I lifted up my head, my neck was abruptly stopped by the steering wheel. I had forgotten I had moved it to the right, to get it down between my legs.

I could see them peering through the window.

"Something looks wrong. Do you think she's fainted? I can't see her face."

"Can you roll down the window?"

No, I can't at the moment. The steering wheel is caught in one of my sweaty neck folds. Please, please, just go away.

Of course, I was just thinking that. And I'm not sure it would have helped. I was sure I looked pretty awful, from where they were standing outside the car.

I tried to get a hand up, so they would know I wasn't expiring or something. It didn't reassure them.

"Hey, I see her hand. Is she trying to tell us something?"

"Maybe we should call 911."

Oh, my God.

I had to do something or the EMTs would come and see my underwear.

OH, MY GOD!

I had fat-girl mothers clucking in my head. They see it in the newspaper, and nod knowingly.

They'd look over at their fat daughter.

"Look at this headline. *'Fat Girl Pried Out of Her Car by Exhausted EMTs'*.

They would read on - out loud of course, so their fat daughters could see their mothers were right all along. The fat-girl mothers had known this would happen.

"After two hours, the 'Jaws of Life' were able to remove the door and roof of the car. They used a winch to pull out the fat girl, who had her enormous neck stuck under the car's steering wheel. As the EMTs pulled her out, her cheap Hawaiian muumuu tore apart, revealing the biggest underpants the extraordinarily good-looking, emergency techs had ever seen. A passer-by with a camera phone caught it all and sent it to YouTube."

I was nothing if not creative in my mental self-abuse, as I waved my arm at the window.

I had to get my head up, so they could see I was okay.

With every bit of strength I could muster, I pushed my neck towards the right. The sweat was actually helping. The steering wheel was getting slick from the water in my neck folds. I also needed to get my head up, because my chest was pushed down into my stomach. It was getting difficult to breathe.

God, don't let me faint. Or if I do, just get it over with and let me die, rather than come back to this horror show that is my life.

With a big sucking sound, my neck came out from under the steering wheel. I came up slowly. I was sure I would black out, if I rose too fast. Not helpful to the concerned citizens outside my window. Except for the guy with the camera phone. I didn't truly believe he was concerned. I bet he was thinking of sending this to one of those comedy programs, that paid for human catastrophes like groin hits, or old people losing their pants in public. They pay a lot of money for good ones. The ones that make us think, "Jesus, that's terrible. Did you see how hard that kid jumped on his balls?" as we laugh hysterically.

Mine would probably win him the top money, and be shown year after year as one of the top humiliating videos of all time.

As I raised my head to look at the people outside the car, I could see them involuntarily take a few steps back from the car window. Their faces looked more frightened than relieved.

I hurried to roll down the window to reassure them. The flab on my arm made an audible plop, as I hit the button that automatically lowers the window.

Crap.

I hadn't turned the key to activate the automatic stuff in the car.

I tried to smile and gesture about the key. By this time, they were backing away.

I guess they knew I was all right.

I looked in the rearview mirror. I knew why they were leaving "the scene of the accident." An appropriate description. I looked like a blowfish with arms.

Fat Girl in the Checkout Line

I definitely had to have a bulimic episode after that. There was a Walgreens's across from the doctor's office.

Where I could have accomplished two things with one stop if that doctor had been compliant. I could have given the pharmacy my prescription for Phentermine, and then enjoyed myself by using at least $50 of my remaining money getting my comfort eats.

Well, I could get my junk food, anyway.

As I walked past the shelves with various household items and over-the-counter medications, I glanced forlornly at all the brown bottles on the white pharmacy shelves. I reached down and picked up some of their 500-milligram caffeine pills, a container of body lotion, and headed for my favorite place in any store – the candy aisle.

For me, it was always a holiday. Whether it was Christmas, Valentine's Day, or Easter when the special candy came out, I was "good to go" on whatever junk food they had to celebrate the holiday. I always had my usual favorites available, too. Sometimes after the holiday was over, they'd have the candy on sale. I loved that, because I could get twice as much.

One after-Christmas sale remains a pleasant memory, when I got "two-for-one" on 1 lb. bags of varied-colored chocolate candies. If they were adding a new color, they'd have lots of those left over. People tend to trust what they know. Stupid really. The chocolate was the same. The shells tasted the same. I guess they had to get attached to the character in the chocolate commercials, to give the new one a try. Or, they emotionally associated with one of the colors. Candy eaters weren't particularly known for their intellects. Except for smart fat girls. We'd buy them, and scarf them down regardless of their colors, if they were on sale.

Sometimes, I'd make a game out of eating them. I'd separate them into different-colored piles. Then, I'd eat all of one color, and then go on to the next until they all were gone. If I was in a hurry or was doing an emotional binge feed, then I'd pour out handfuls, and thrust them in my mouth until the bag was gone.

When I went to check out, I'd do a variation of the act I used in McDonald's. Nothing worse than seeing a fat girl with a full basket of candy, sale or not.

I put the lotion next to the cashier first. I'd then start talking.

"Boy, with heat like this, this lotion was at the top of my list."

I'd take a piece of paper from my purse I had written the day before. It had names on it, and a place to make a checkmark next to each name. I would ask the cashier if I could borrow a pen. They usually had one or two of the generic kind, for those customers who paid with something other than cash.

I made sure I always had enough cash. I had learned my lesson about what can happen if there was a problem with their computer, and the credit card machine went down. I didn't want to have to wait. The time had to be as short as possible, so people shopping wouldn't happen to glance up, and see the fat girl with the ten pounds of chocolates and crème-filled cakes waiting at the register. I could pay quickly with cash, and leave before anyone took notice of me.

When she would give me a pen, it would focus her attention on what I was doing. As I lifted the bags of chocolate out of the basket, I would look at my list, with the pen poised. I would talk loudly enough, so that anyone in line behind me could also hear:

"These are Jenny's." I'd make a checkmark on the paper.

"Bobby wanted two bags of these." Checkmark made.

This would continue, until all the bags were checked out.

"Well, it looks like I got everyone's."

I'd fold the paper over, put it back into my purse and return her pen.

I'd have the cash in my hand. More than was needed. I knew to plan in advance.

I tried to wait until there was no one in line to check out. It didn't occur very often. The fat girl trying to buy her comfort food would be by herself for a fraction of a second, before half the store decided to check out. We were truly cursed. God must have been bored, looked down, saw a fat girl, and lined her up like a carnival target for humiliation.

It happened to me several times. I learned if I didn't have cash, I didn't get my junk food at that particular time. This is how it was the last time I forgot to bring cash. The voices would start behind me:

"Why has the line stopped?"

"Their computers are down."

"Oh no, the one time I'm in a hurry."

"Does that person have lots to check out?"

All twelve people in line craned their necks, to see who was waiting to check out.

The fat girl is silently kicking herself for not bringing cash.

It hurts less if I use third person when remembering. I have a lot of bad memories of my life as a fat girl, as you have already discovered if you have gotten this far in the book. You have read many third-person narratives I've recounted. All true. Not one made-up conversation or enhanced description.

The people in line were less than kind. They chatted among themselves, as if she was deaf. .

They looked at the bags of chocolate and packaged cakes, spread across the entire counter in front of the register:

"My God, that's a lot of candy."

"She must have cleaned out the clearance shelves all by herself."

"What could she possibly do with all that chocolate?"

They stepped out of line with one foot, so they could get a better look.

"Wow, I wouldn't think she'd want to add any more weight."

"Jeez, you'd think she'd put some nutritional things in there."

There were the requisite number of thins in line to embarrass her. They traveled in pairs. They were louder than the rest.

"That's really awful. "

"Yeah, grossness personified."

"How could anyone let themselves go like that?"

The other line members nodded in agreement, like bobble heads at a baseball game.

Don't they think she has any feelings?

She knew any fat girls who were thinking of checking out, moved back into the aisles out of the line of fire. They pretended they were totally concentrating on the thirty types of deodorant in front of them. They would separate. They knew not to stand next to each other. One would move as fast as possible to the other side of the store. You especially don't want to be with another fat girl, if one is under attack. Once the attackers got going, they could be next, if they were hanging around near the massacre. There's no sisterhood with fat girls. You're on your own, if you get noticed. You made the mistake; you should have planned better. Don't look for us to help you. They'll turn on us, too. Who needs that today?

I knew I wouldn't get any help from anyone. I was a fat girl.

From that final time when I didn't bring cash, I would check the cash in my wallet over and over before I went into a store.

After the disappointing doctor's appointment, I was ready to do my act in Walgreen's. I had prepared my fake list before taking off for my doctor's visit. I figured I'd give them the prescription at the pharmacy, then get my junk food. Now, since I didn't have to wait for the Phentermine, I selected my bags and packages and put them in the brown carrying basket. There weren't any sales, so I figured this would cost me about $25 to $30. I'd still have some left for another co-pay. I could probably coax some money out of Mother to pay for the prescription I'd get from a new doctor I'd pick later, after I binged and purged at home.

When I got to the register, cash in hand, I performed my dramatic scene, picked up the shopping bag full of my binge food, and carried it to the car.

Mother asked me how the appointment had gone. I told her he wanted me to get some tests. I'd need some money for the co-pays for tomorrow.

She went to get her purse. Over her shoulder she asked:

"Does he know what caused you to put on all that weight? You had done so well with your diet at school. Did something cause you to eat too much again over there?"

"No, he wasn't sure. Maybe it's my thyroid. I read it can stimulate appetite, if it's not working like it should."

"Well, maybe the tests will show something."

I doubt it, since I'm not having any, I thought to myself.

If I did have tests, I wouldn't want to know the results. Since I was going back to bulimia, I knew I would be fine. It had saved me before. I just needed to get the amphetamine, to get things done properly.

I went to my room, opened my laptop, and searched for the nearest Urgent Care clinic. If I couldn't con a regular doctor (who wanted to improve my health, for God's sake*)*, then I'd pay an exorbitant price to a Physician's Assistant who had a pharmacy right down the hall. Other bulimics and drug users suggested that, when I typed in "Where can I get my amphetamine without a hassle?" on the Internet sites for bulimics who were perfecting their techniques.

I wrote down the address, put it in my purse, made a new list of names, and poured the contents of my haul at Walgreen's on the floor. As I sorted them into groups, I felt tired but relieved. It was like returning to a former lover. Bulimia would show me the affection I didn't get from the world as a fat girl. It knew what to do to make me happy. I reached into the first pile. I smiled. It was one of those packages with two large peanut butter cookies. As I ate, I thought back to the moment when I became a food addict, my substitution for love.

First Love

Because of my father's health condition, Mother didn't buy junk food. But she was obsessed about being loved at work. She provided all kinds of sweets to satisfy my cravings.

Her "people pleaser" behavior would serve me well, as I began my journey to food addiction.

When I was a kid and starting on my fat life, I'd have little methods to get what I needed from Mother's candy supply she used for her "Love me" cakes.

One of my favorites was the bag of baking chocolate bits she stored in the cupboards. She'd have bags of white chocolate, as well as the **Hershey** flavored. They were like miniature spherical kisses. At the top of each one, the candy machine would finish each one with a little chocolate curl. Sometimes, I'd bite the curl off, and let it roam around in my mouth for a while before I'd finish the rest.

She'd shop on Thursdays for her overnight baking. I'd help her carry in the groceries, if I was home from school in time. I could feel the bumpy packages through the brown paper sacks, if I squeezed hard enough. Not too hard, though, or when Mother emptied out the groceries, the candy bags would have burst open, and be at the bottom of the sack in one big multi-colored mound. Mother's OCD would balk at things mixed together like that. She had her recipes that she followed without deviation. There wasn't a little pinch of this or a small bit of that in our meals.

On my kid plate, I had separate sections for each food. I'd have a fit if they got mixed somehow. Until I had everything in its proper place, I wouldn't eat anything. Bulimia helped my OCD compulsion, because I would grab lots of different stuff and cram them in. I wouldn't keep them in my mouth for long. I wasn't savoring the flavors. I got the soda going, so they'd go down, and I'd have the next load ready to go in. It wasn't the food; it was the feeling I got bingeing on the food. Of course, the guilt would follow with the purging ritual. But after I had done both, it was an indescribable sensation. My mind said my stomach was empty, so I wouldn't gain weight. My emotions had been fed by the food that loved me. It never criticized me; called me names, made fun of me, or rejected me. It was my friend. It loved me unconditionally. I could do no wrong.

Mother was careful about when she baked, because my father was a diabetic. It was the adult kind. He was diagnosed in his late forties. He loved sweets, especially pecan or coconut pie. Mother tried to make him adhere to a diabetic diet, but she noticed when she made goodies during the week for Fridays, some of her pie would be missing.

"What happened to my pecan pie? There are two big slices missing."

She would glare at my father. She knew my favorite was lemon meringue, so I wasn't the thief.

My father would stare at the floor like a little kid.

"I just wanted a couple of slices. They won't hurt me."

"Your blood sugar is going to go through the roof."

When he was tested that week, the doctor said he'd have to start him on insulin

So, Mother began her baking on Thursday nights for Friday office take ins. He couldn't sneak any anymore, because she would bake them late, and have them in the car by the time he got up.

My father was a southerner who loved to eat. Before he was diagnosed, we'd have fried something every night for dinner. It would be followed by sugar-laden desserts. Nowadays, his cholesterol would have competed with his blood sugar for which was worse. He died of heart disease and advanced diabetes. At the end, he couldn't feel his feet because the blood flow was so bad. He had high blood pressure, too. He didn't survive his second open-heart surgery for heart grafts. He was only 62. I often wondered why he didn't drink. I thought it was because of Mother. I found out after he died, that his father had been an alcoholic.

Mother's kitchen routine was pretty well established when I did my early-morning raids. She'd lay everything out for a particular recipe. Then, she would proceed step by step, until she had her cookies, cakes or pies baked and cooling on the kitchen counter.

Since I was getting pudgy, she wouldn't let me have any leftovers in the bowls. The smells would drive me wild at night, as I heard her mixing and pouring. The sound of the oven opening and closing would be like a dinner bell in my brain.

She'd finally come upstairs to get some shut-eye, until she had to go to work.

I'd wait an extra half-hour, just to be sure she was asleep. I had socks on so my feet didn't make any sound, as I took the stairs two at a time. I had a small flashlight in the bedside drawer, that I brought downstairs with me for my kitchen raids. No room lights could be turned on. I sometimes used the flashlight late at night for a binge-and purge session. I made sure I always had a spare set of batteries for it.

At the third step from the bottom, I'd pause and close my eyes. I'd enjoy the smells coming from the cooling cookies and pies on their metal plates.

I'd open my eyes, and it would be like Christmas morning. Usually, the whole counter would be filled. I loved peanut butter cookies that were still warm from the oven. They were so soft. Sometimes, if I didn't let them cool enough, they'd break apart in my hands. Her office mates liked them, too, so at almost every baking, there would be at least three batches.

Since Mother was a perfectionist, the cookies would be lined up on the long flat trays. If the majority of them had four in each row, I knew if I took from those she'd see right away, as she was putting tin foil over each bunch on the decorative plates she used. The symmetry would be off. I had to hope that some of the rows had five or more in them. I was lucky most of the time. She always made more than was necessary, to feed the entire office twice over.

She didn't bring anything home, though. It was dangerous for my father, and I was gaining too much weight as it was.

And she could be loved even more, if she had leftovers for them to take home. She'd even wrap them in tin foil she brought to work. If it was a pie, she would tell them to keep the pie container. She would slide the cakes and cookies onto disposable plates in the little coffee kitchen at the back of the office, before the office closed for the day. Her ceramic plates and trays would be washed and later taken to the car, after everyone had gotten their goodies to take home.

Mother with her baking was as OCD as I was. When I was close enough to the kitchen counter to smell the food, I'd turn on my flashlight and shine it over the wonderful panorama of baked treats she had made for the office. Everything was grouped according to its category. Three cakes on the far end of the counter. Two pies closer in next to them. Finally, the trays of cookies nestling close to the wall at the other end of the counter.

I'd first look to see if she'd left any bags of candy under the shelves near the refrigerator. She was meticulous so there weren't any, unless she was particularly tired and thought she'd clean up in the morning. I was really excited, if there were new bags of baking chocolate. I could poke a hole big enough for one to get out, at one corner of the bottom of the bag. There was usually some space at the top in each bag. I just had to be careful that the level didn't go down too much. I'd start with squeezing gently on the bag, until one curly-topped tiny kiss dropped into my hand. I'd put it in my mouth and suck on it until it was gone, as I surveyed the cookies, cakes, and pies in front of me.

The pies were tricky to steal from. If the crust broke off, I couldn't fix it like I could the cakes. The fruit pies were the ones I could get the most from. Mother would have put those flour ribbons across them before she put them in the oven, to keep the fruit from running over the sides of the tins. There would still be some leaking through around them. After I laid the baking chocolate bag gently on the counter, I'd take my left forefinger and carefully scrape the bulging fruit off. I had to watch out I didn't use too much pressure. I didn't want to break into the crust, or cause a crack in any of the flour ribbons. The scraping didn't affect the appearance of the pie, and I'd get the delicious overflow. The biggest glob was often at the top. It would look like colored fruit lava ready to erupt. I could use two fingers on those tops. I'd curl the first two fingers of my right hand, scoop them off and pop them in my mouth. I had to lick off both hands' fingers after each pie. Since I was using the same fingers, I couldn't have any trace of the one pie on them, when I took the scrapings and top off another one. The fruit colors couldn't mix, or her eye would be drawn to the mixed-color combinations before she wrapped them up.

I'd go back to my tiny kisses, after I had finished the overflow fruit on each pie. I'd push out another miniature chocolate and put it in my mouth to suck, while I went on to the next pie. By the time the chocolate had dissolved in my mouth, I'd be ready with my scrape or scoop of pie to eat.

The cakes were next. If she had swirled the frosting with a knife, I couldn't run my finger around them like I could if they had flat frosting covering them. When she'd make a lot of cakes for special occasions, I'd have at least two that had the frosting I could steal from. I could even fill any holes I might make, because some sides had more frosting than the others.

I had the same procedure for the kisses and the cakes. I still shook only one out each time, because I was going on to the cookies. For each cookie, I'd eat one tiny kiss. There were many more cookies than the cakes and pies.

Mother had made two different kinds. One tray was layered with white chocolate cookies. The other cookies were peanut butter. I counted the rows. The majority of the rows had three. Yeah! I immediately went to the rows that had more. I took two paper towels from the towel holder, and laid them side-by-side on the counter next to the cookie sheets.

On one, I put the five extra from one tray. On the other, I put four that were overflow from the other. That meant I could eat nine more candy kisses.

I couldn't use the spatulas to remove them from the sheet. It might make too much noise. I would stop every five minutes to listen. Just in case one of them came downstairs to get a drink.

Sometimes, in the back of my mind as I was gorging, I would think about being found out.

Maybe I want to get caught.

They'd be surprised and a little disgusted. But that would turn into guilt and concern. They'd be panicked about losing me. They'd want to help me. They would get me to a doctor right away. Maybe load me in the car right then and there, and take me to the local hospital's Emergency Room. They would get me help, because they loved me. Was this a way to get their affection? Was that why I was doing this?

At thirteen, I couldn't do a psych evaluation on myself. I just wanted my parents to care about me. Even a negative response was better than nothing. I would eat, until they noticed how fat I was getting. The more they were disappointed, dismayed and angry; the more I would eat. It was a simple solution to being ignored. I would get their attention. If they got after me about my weight, I'd know how much they loved me.

As I got fatter, they got more critical and upset. It was working. At thirteen, I had figured out how to get what I needed from my parents. I was proud of myself.

I put big pieces of the cookies in my mouth. I grinned like an idiot.

I followed this plan for several years. It was flawless. I had gained a hefty amount of weight. I was good at becoming fat. Straight As in school, where I was friendless and abused. Constantly berated at home, and getting fat for love. I was perfection.

And then I found my lifelong friends that made me complete. Bulimia and phentermine. My perfectionism and OCD loved these addictions. I couldn't have found ones that fit me better

As I relived my first foray into food addiction, I was pleased to see my food piles had diminished greatly. I could eat without being aware of it. Bingeing was as natural as could be for me.

My stomach was extended and aching, so I gathered the remnants of my comfort food, and put them in my hiding spots in my room. The bathroom was next. I was looking forward to getting that feeling of contentment back. I started to purge.

Chapter 11

No Help at All

My visit to the Urgent Care clinic was a bust. I thought I had him. He was falling for my story. The guy was going to come through for me. He didn't want to run any tests. He was writing me a prescription.

Damn.

He wrote it for Prozac. I guess he decided I was fat, because I was depressed. It should have been the other way around. Prozac made you eat more, because you weren't depressed, anymore. I even knew that.

I'm fat, for crissakes. Give me something to make me stop eating. Give me my phentermine.

Nope. I get a stupid anti-depressant, that will make me tired while I eat.

Crap and double crap.

The hell with the medical establishment. I would get what I needed some other way. I needed money. Fine. I would find a job I could do at home. I didn't want to be seen in public on a professional level, until I lost the weight I had gained. If I made enough to pay my mother back, give them some money for rent and food, and pay my credit card payment each month, I would be all set. I could still borrow Mother's car to get my binge haul. They didn't expect me to socialize. I didn't need clothes, until I dropped the pounds. This was going to work out. I just needed to find a job I could do through the Internet.

It turned out to be easy. With my college background, I could sell textbooks online to universities. The pay was good.

My parents were relieved I'd be occupied. They expected me to move out, once I got a permanent position in the fall. When I lost the fat, I could go to interviews. Perfect.

Until I paid my card down, I couldn't use it for ordering phentermine online. Simple. Get another credit card. While I was waiting for it, my bulimia would come through for me. Mother was still doing her baking thing. I could get my junk food until I got paid.

The new credit card arrived in a week. It had a $5,000 limit. I was ecstatic. I ordered phentermine from six online pharmacies, and paid the fee for Overnight shipping on all of them.

Since I was home most of the time, I would be there to sign for the packages. I told my parents I had ordered some high-powered vitamins to take while I was dieting.

When the first bottle of phentermine arrived, I decided to take more than the prescribed dosage. I had ordered full strength again. Five more brown bottles with 30 capsules each were on their way.

Since I was going to be low on funds for a while, I decided to alter my food intake. I knew the phentermine would cut my appetite, but I still needed the bulimia for the feeling it gave me. So I put my OCD into gear, and chose one thing to eat per day. I would throw it up, anyway, but the calories wouldn't be as massive. I looked in the cupboard to see what we had already in the house. That way, I wouldn't raise any suspicions about what I was doing, if Mother was already buying the product.

I chose cheese crackers. They were portable around the house. They had family-sized boxes. Mother wouldn't care, because they said "cheese" on the box. My father was allowed a box of cheese crackers per week. They would fill me up, if I ate a box at a time. They weren't messy, and I didn't have to hide them. Perfect.

It took me a couple of glorious days to finish my junk food. I was also taking three phentermine a day. My appetite was waning. My heartbeat was abnormally fast, even for an amphetamine. Risky, but what the hell. I'd rather be dead than fat.

After I had purged the last of my stash, I went downstairs, grabbed the box of cheese crackers, and took it to my room. That evening, I finished most of the box while I was watching television in my room. I made sure to leave some, in case my father wanted some, and the box was missing.

I purged just fine on them. Some came back up in lumps, but after vomiting them in the first retching, the others came up a few at a time. It took only five minutes to get just one food back up. I liked that. Less noise and less cleanup.

On my first trip to the store to get them, I bought five family-sized ones and two smaller ones. I went to two different stores, since that seemed like a lot for one purchase. I didn't want to get noticed.

Thus began my regime of one meal a day with a box of cheese crackers. I always put one of the small boxes in the cupboard, so there would be one there for my father. When Mother would buy a box, I 'd take the one I put in there back to my room.

With the three phentermines and the restricted diet, I was losing about 5 pounds a week. I didn't count the first ten pounds as fat loss, because it was water weight I was losing.

I could have done the whole three months with the crackers, but I thought Mother might notice. I ate the cheese crackers one day, and alternated the next with jars of dry roasted peanuts. I could shop at one store, since I was buying two products. My father could eat a limited amount of those, too.

The peanuts were even a better purge food than the crackers. They were smaller, and the stomach acid dissolved them faster. Not many clumps came up.

At the end of a month, I had lost almost 25 pounds. I had 35 still to lose in two months. Things looked good. My plan was working.

I didn't eat anything but the cheese crackers and the peanuts. My parents didn't ask about my diet. I had usually eaten in my room instead of with them, so it wasn't unusual for them not to see me for meals. I was losing weight, so they didn't criticize my appearance. Mother thought I was getting multi-vitamins frequently through the mail, so I wouldn't get sick from dieting.

I noticed some changes after the first month, I hadn't seen before. The bulimic episodes tired me out. I'd have my energy back with the phentermines, though. One balanced the other. But now, I was tired all the time. It was harder to concentrate. It would take me twice as long to complete an order. I put off making business contacts online, because I had to adopt a different persona with clients. I couldn't seem to get up the energy to dialog with them, to sell the company's textbooks.

I had post-it notes on all four sides of my computer, to keep me on schedule. Sometimes, I wouldn't feel the urge to eat, so I didn't. I was down to half a box of crackers and a half jar of peanuts. I'd forget to eat.

I couldn't sleep, even though I was exhausted. The third phentermine at night kept me awake. When I did lie down, my heart palpitations were more noticeable. I thought my heart would leap out of my chest, at times

I wasn't even 25 years old, but I felt like I was 50. Maybe it was harder to bounce back, now that I was older. That could account for the symptoms. I wasn't scared or worried. I had been bulimic and amphetamine-addicted for years. They were my lifestyle.

It would probably be temporary, like any reactions I'd had in the past. I certainly didn't want to tell my parents, or have them find out on their own. I had done such a brilliant job of hiding my addictions. And I definitely didn't want to see a doctor.

No such luck.

I had forgotten about the yearly appointments Mother made for all of us with the family physician and dentist. When we didn't want to go, she'd say:

"It's better to catch things early, than wait until something becomes a big problem."

Close Call

Mother reminded me the day before my appointment with our family doctor. I thought of a dozen reasons why I couldn't go, but her OCD loved rigid appointment schedules. She'd argue until we got so irritated, we'd agree just to get her off our backs.

"That's how we found out about your father. At one of his annual checkups."

I did some meditation exercises to lower my blood pressure before I left. I didn't take my morning phentermine dose, so my hands wouldn't shake. I had become quite impatient and irritable. More than I remembered from my last time with phentermine.

I'm getting used to it again, and I've increased the daily dosage. That would explain the symptoms I'm having.

I had figured it out. Good.

I hadn't been in a fat cycle when he had seen me - ever. It would have been too embarrassing. He would have been disappointed in me. I had known him since I was a kid. He liked me when I was skinny. I couldn't face his disapproval.

He'd want to know why. He'd think like the rest of the world, that I was a lazy, fat slob who couldn't control her eating. Fortunately, I was always in one of my thin cycles when my yearly appointment arrived. It was just luck.

I knew my weight was really up since the last time I had seen him. It had been my checkup before I left for my job in Hawaii, so I was really skinny due to my toast-diet soda starvation diet. In fact, I remember he had commented on that.

"You've lost quite a bit of weight."

He was peering at me through his horn-rimmed glasses. I uncrossed my legs, so one wasn't hidden by the other. That had become a habit. It was one of my OCD checks on my state of being thin. I had jeans on, so he couldn't see my bony knees. But I had forgotten about my face and arms. I quickly turned over my forearms, so they were face down on the chair arms. If he looked closely enough, he'd see the veins. They were big and long. My skin wasn't thick enough to cover them. I was pretty sure my body was eating muscle at this point. I never worried, 'though. What's a little muscle compared to being thin? I knew my priorities.

My face had a hollowed-out look. I should have loaded on the makeup, and put on a really red lipstick to make my lips look larger. I had put my hair behind my ears, instead of around my face. I reached up, and casually moved it towards my cheeks and neck. I twirled a strand in my fingers, as if that was an unconscious habit I had when I was talking. I leaned back in the chair, to give my shirt more room to show. Leaning forward had made it taut against my chest and waist.

"I've been pretty busy and a little stressed getting ready to leave for Hawaii. I haven't been there before. The pictures in the books I'm reading show lots of gorgeous places. Have you been there?"

I knew how busy he was. I thought if I could turn his attention away from my weight, he'd go on with the examination. It worked. He looked back down to my chart.

I hadn't looked forward to having my checkup. I was concerned about the medical parts of it. I could lie on the update paperwork, but the blood pressure cuff and stethoscope were my enemies.

I was kind of looking forward to seeing what my weight was, 'though. I had been on my starvation diet for almost two months. I knew the medical scale would be accurate. For better or worse.

"Okay, if you'd hop up on the scale, we'll get your weight."

I quickly removed my shoes, and set them and my purse next to the scale. I stepped on. I didn't close my eyes this time. I watched her move the metal tabs – 120, 125, 130, 140 *Stop! Stop!* 145, 150 - the heavy metal bar fell deafeningly into the slot.

Crap. I'm closing my eyes.

I couldn't stand to see it cumbersomely rise from that notch and go on.

Hell, I thought I was doing so well.

I had thought my cheekbones were becoming visible, and I felt some ribs when I pushed down hard on my chest. Maybe my fat cells weren't cooperating. I thought it would take longer this time, but I had upped the amphetamine, and cut out the junk food completely. Maybe the crackers and peanuts had too much fat, even though I was down to half a box and half a jar. I threw up as soon as I ate my fill. Maybe the gods weren't on my side this time. I was pretty sure God was indifferent. Maybe my luck had run out. I was destined to be fat forever.

My depression was deepening every second I was on that damn scale. I couldn't even hope the scale was wrong. Medical scales are never wrong. In one of my dieting cycles, after I had found out about phentermine, I brought my weight scale out of the closet, and put it in my bathroom. After every purge, I'd eagerly step on. Usually, fat girls have scales with spider webs on them from non-use, if they have scales at all. If you couldn't see how fat you were, it was a way to avoid facing a fat-girl truth. You could still make believe you had some right to happiness; you were still worthy of love. Pitiful delusions.

The medical assistant was talking to me, but I hadn't been listening. I opened my eyes, and the number was right in front of me. I had blocked out the clicks from 150 on. It had stopped at 154! I had lost over 30 pounds, but I couldn't show that to her. She was new and didn't know me. I felt I had to explain the difference she would see in my chart, when she recorded my weight today.

"It's a little up from the last time I was here. It was all that Hawaiian rich food."

Her eyes moved away from the scale.

"Were you over there for a vacation"

"I got a job there right out of college. I was so lucky. I've been living there for two years. I just retuned last week."

"Is it as beautiful as they say?"

"More. The beaches are so white they hurt your eyes."

She was now leading me to an examination room. I had slipped on my shoes, and picked up my purse as we were talking.

"Let's get your blood pressure."

I mentally slowed my breathing, while she puffed up the cuff.

She didn't say anything, as she listened for the pauses through the stethoscope she had placed next to the cuff.

As she was removing it, I wanted to know what it showed. Was it too high? Was it going to be a problem?

I decided not to ask. If it was a little high, that would be okay. If it was sky high, I was going to have major issues with the doctor.

She didn't say anything, as she jotted the number in the chart. She smiled, and said as she was leaving:

"The doctor will be in to see you in a few minutes."

Yes!

I had dodged another medical bullet.

I heard her put my file in the plastic holder next to the exam room door.

My doctor came in ten minutes later. He took the stool next to a small counter, where he put my chart. While he was reading it, I perused the pictures of healthy organs stapled to the wall above the counter.

Mine probably didn't look like those. I couldn't see them, anyway, so it was not a big deal. I was only in my twenties. I had years to get my system back in shape, *after* I was permanently thin.

He wanted to do a thorough workup, because he wanted to make sure everything was fine. I took the paperwork, thanked him and left.

When I got home, I told Mother things went well. I put the medical lab forms in my desk. I realized later I should have followed through. They would have caught the blood infection and the early osteoporosis.

As the weeks passed into the final month of summer, the physiological changes I had noticed earlier, escalated. I had some new signs, too, that my body was under siege. I had deprived it of nutrients for a long time. It was payback time.

When I had lost all the weight I gained in Hawaii, and an extra 10 pounds just to be sure I wouldn't get fat again, there was visible deterioration that was hard to ignore. My hair was thinning and brittle. The nervousness I had with phentermine had caused me to peel away the layers of skin near my fingernails. It was something I did constantly, without thinking about it. The skin near my thumbnail especially took a beating. It was raw and bleeding all the time. I put a Band-Aid on it, when it became too painful to use as it was. The Band-Aid kept me from worsening the situation, too. I would have dug at it, until it was down through several skin layers.

I found I really had to control my emotions. They were intensified. Irritability frequently became angry outbursts with anyone who seemed incompetent. That pretty much meant anyone I came in contact with. I cussed out other drivers for their stupidity on the road. I became obstreperous, if I didn't get what I wanted immediately from anyone. Words came out of my mouth without thinking. And they usually weren't kind. I became what I despised the most in society – intolerant, judgmental and hateful. I was worse than the worse thin. My psychological state reflected the years of bulimia and drug abuse, along with the physical manifestations. Unfortunately, more bad news was on its way.

My dentist's receptionist called to confirm the appointment Mother had set up for me. I had avoided the dentist more than any other doctor. My extensive knowledge of what might happen with chronic bulimic behavior, included an in-depth description of the deterioration of the gums and teeth. I had seen him before I left for Hawaii. Mother, again with her OCD scheduling of checkup appointments, had fixed it so I had to see him once more.

I hadn't paid much attention to that area. My purging ritual included brushing, flossing and mouthwash. I told her I didn't need to go. But she was insistent as usual. It was one more thing she could check off her list of things that needed to be done.

When I started my eating disorder, I didn't pay attention to how much sugar I was taking in through the candy I constantly ate. At fourteen, my yearly checkup showed I had 12 cavities. Mother was embarrassed. What kind of parent lets her kid get 12 cavities? It took weeks of painful dental work and quite a bit of money, to get my teeth repaired. I was *persona non grata* at home, too. Mother even threatened to watch me while I brushed my teeth. I convinced her she didn't need to do that. For a while, I showed her my teeth and gums after each brushing. Except for the purge brushing, of course.

After that unpleasant experience with my dentist, I altered my quantity of candy. I still ate bags of it, but I tried to spread it out over the bingeing periods. I was eating plenty of other junk food, so I didn't feel deprived. The dentist had finished my treatment by putting a protective coating on my teeth. I hoped it would help keep me from getting an exorbitant number of cavities again.

Even though I hadn't seen a dentist for two years, I thought I'd be okay. My roommate and I feasted on pasta and chips more than anything else. Oddly, I switched to diet soda to wash the pounds of food down my throat. In some weird, rationalizing way, drinking diet soda made it okay to consume as much junk food as I wanted.

It was like checking my wrist size. I thought if I didn't drink soda with all that sugar in it, I wouldn't be as fat. Of course, I was throwing down full three-course meals as much as I could. And they never included fruits and vegetables.

Irrational fat-girl attitude. We have a multitude of ways to delude ourselves. Goes with the territory.

Final Call

This time, on my post-Hawaii visit, I had brushed my teeth, flossed for all I was worth, and did several mouthfuls of mouthwash before I left for the dentist. I was really seeing the dental hygienist. She would take the x-rays and clean my teeth. The dentist just popped in at the end of the appointment, to do a final cursory check. But I almost didn't see him at all this time.

Sometimes, if I stretched my mouth to accommodate my bulimic fingers and the food coming back up, I would develop "mouth slits." At each end would be a cut, several inches long. They especially appeared if my skin was dry. It is a common result from the loss of elasticity and texture in a bulimic's skin. If I didn't put some antibiotic cream all over my mouth, I would get cracks in my lips and slits at the sides of my mouth.

I hadn't noticed that I had some that were healing, when I kept my dentist appointment. The dental hygienist did, though. As she approached my mouth to take a look after putting on her gloves, she stopped and backed away.

"What are those on your mouth?"

Crap. Think fast

"Oh, those. My skin gets dry with this weather. If I don't put lotion on my face, I'll get these things."

I was pretty safe with the weather excuse. It's almost always hot and dry in Arizona. I held my breath.

She nodded and came over to do a mouth sweep to look for abnormalities.

She finished her finger sweep, and got her tray set up for the cleaning procedure.

Well, at least I didn't have mouth cancer.

I still wasn't home free, though.

At the end of the cleaning, she flosses. My gums started to bleed.

Damn.

I hadn't thought about brushing at the gum level. When I "purged flossed," I was only looking for bits of food on the string. I didn't floss using the mirror above the counter, either. I avoided looking at myself after a purge. Much shame and guilt.

She gave me a lecture on the dangers of letting my gums go. For one thing, the bacteria from the gums can infect the lining of the heart. That didn't sound good.

"That sounds awful. I'll be more careful when I brush, so I do it at the gum line."

She smiled, and left to get the dentist. He came in, and did his "twenty-second" check. He always smelled like peppermint.

"Looks good. I'll take a look at the x-rays. If I see anything to worry about, I'll give you a call."

"Sounds good to me."

I was handed my new toothbrush and a container of floss.

"See you next year."

I was out the door with a huge sigh of relief. That had been a close call.

Et Tu, Paranoia?

The doctor and dentist visits were eye opening about my physical degeneration. Incipient diseases were not going to influence me, though. Nothing would make me sacrifice my thinness. My brain said so. It was saying other things, too. I was my mother's child.

Mother was high strung. That was the penultimate excuse my father used to explain her dysfunctional behavior. It had the connotation of being complimentary. If you were high strung, you had extraordinary sensitivity and intelligence. So if you were irrational, temperamental, depressed, and even suicidal, it was because the world didn't understand you. It wasn't your fault. You should "get a pass" on "losing it." You didn't really mean what you said. Since you were so intelligent and misunderstood, it was almost expected you'd have moments of desperation and sadness. We all should understand.

Nope.

Mother was passive-aggressive; another component of her mental illness.

My mother hated herself for her self-sacrifice to get love. She had a grudge against a world that should have recognized her abilities. If she raised her voice at work, or offered an opinion, she'd immediately go into her passive, self-critical, self-denigrating role. She would say she didn't really think what she had said was relevant, if her colleagues or boss said something different. She would say she didn't know enough to give her advice.

Mother lowered her shoulders, plastered a smile on her face, and twisted her hands, when she would meekly engage in conversation. She looked like a whipped dog. I saw her do this with the neighbors, with sales people, with waitresses, with people who had made a mistake and were the ones in the wrong. She had assumed this persona as a girl, growing up in the oppressive environment her father had raised her in. Be obedient, be afraid, and be quiet. The cellar was waiting for bad girls. She would lose her job. She would be disliked; worse – unloved.

"Are you sure I can't get that for you?"

"Of course, I'll watch your house while you're on vacation. Did you want me to water your plants, take your dogs for walks, get your mail?"

They would offer to pay her.

She'd wave her hands and say:

"No, no. I couldn't take anything for that. I'd be glad to do it for you."

"Can I get you anything while I'm out shopping?"

They would go get their purses.

"Oh, don't worry about it. You can pay me later."

"No, no. I'm sure it was my fault."

"Yes, you're right. I must have done that. I don't have my head screwed on today."

If some of her treats hadn't been touched an hour after she came in, she would ask several people:

"Was something wrong? That was a new recipe. I probably didn't put enough flour in the batter."

The words "I'm sorry" were the first she would utter, before and after a conversation in public. What did she know? She was a secretary. Everybody must be more intelligent than the "office gofer." She was so grateful when they said they liked her. But she implied she was unworthy of their appreciation of her skills. She was sure nobody listened or took her seriously. Why should they? She regretted opening her mouth in the first place. She hoped she hadn't said the wrong thing, hurt someone's feelings, hadn't shown how much she was grateful for what they said or did. She was a nervous wreck at work, trying to be the ultimate people-pleaser.

At home, it was her aggressive personality that predominated. All that pent-up rage over how she was mistreated, came out as soon as she walked through the door.

"Do you know what happened today?"

I wasn't expected to answer. It was the lead-in for her rant.

"I typed his letter perfectly. He made the mistake."

"Nobody said anything when *I* did their work, so they could catch up."

"I bet the new girl is going to get that promotion, even though I've been there fifteen years. I can take dictation and type letters faster than anyone in that office."

"That sales lady must think we're poor. She showed us the clearance rack first thing."

"They gave me the wrong salad. She didn't even notice"

"Those neighbors across from us are going to want me to take care of their house, while they're on some expensive vacation somewhere. Don't they think I have better things to do with my time? I have my own house and family."

Once she was tired of talking about her woes at work, she would start in on me.

"Did you do what I asked you to do?"

"What happened in school today? Did you make any friends?"

"What am I going to do with you?"

I took my social cues from Mother on how to think about the people she knew. If she liked them one day; she didn't like them the next. If we loved her and wanted her love, we would feel the same about them. It was emotional blackmail. We were against her, too, if we didn't believe, or we questioned what she said about her co-workers, her boss, neighbors, or strangers.

Someone would look at her, as if she was unimportant. She'd want to hurt them before they hurt her. She was obsessed with the idea people were using her, deceiving her, lying to her. When she'd drink, the paranoia would become exacerbated. The world was against her; it never gave her a chance, and she would hold a lifelong grudge against it. It was not her fault; it was everybody else's, when something didn't end up the way she wanted it. Of course, the way she wanted it changed daily, sometimes hourly, if she was drunk. She was never sure if people liked her. With her father's perspective about her abilities, she knew you had to earn love. She didn't believe anybody really cared about her or understood her.

Since she couldn't expose her true feelings to the outside world, we were the ones who had to listen to her, since no one else did. We owed her that; she had given up her own life for ours. The unhappier she was; the more shame and guilt we felt. It was our fault she was miserable and angry. It was worse because we were supposed to love her, no matter what. Look what she had done for us; what she sacrificed.

If her father called, we were in for a terrible couple of days with her. On the phone with him, she talked like a child. I was surprised. She had told me countless times, how he had never let her be what she wanted to be. Her drinking was his fault. He never showed he loved her. She was never good enough for him. I expected her to tell him what she felt. Although she was far away from him, she was still fearful and submissive.

"Yes, Father, I will do that right away."

"I should have called or written sooner. I'm sorry you had to call me."

"We'll try to get down there to see you. Yes, I know Mother is not feeling well. I know it's hard on both of you."

"Yes, I will, Father, as soon as I get off the phone. I'm so sorry you both are not feeling well. You're right. If I was a good daughter, I wouldn't have made you have to call me. I promise I'll call every Sunday. Goodbye, Father."

When she'd finish the phone call, she'd immediately go to the refrigerator to get a tall drink from the container with her vodka. She'd brood about her conversation with her father.

"I should have told him what I really felt."

I'd make the mistake of asking her why she hadn't. It seemed clear to me she wanted to berate him for what he had done to her life. She'd say she couldn't do it. He had made her so indecisive and meek, she couldn't even tell him the truth.

But we would know how she felt. After a couple more tall ones, she'd really get going.

"What a bastard."

"He never loved me."

"Look what he's done. It's all his fault, the mean son of a bitch."

So I was supposed to hate him, too. My relations with my grandparents were abnormal, to say the least. If I talked with him when he called, Mother would watch me like a hawk, to make sure I'd tell him how much I loved him, and appreciated all he had done for Mother. She'd make me write letters, send holiday cards, and draw pictures for him. She'd always check to see I had been properly thankful for being his granddaughter, in whatever I wrote or drew. I had to put "I love you" on everything I sent. After she was satisfied with the amount of affection I had been required to show, she'd send them off to him.

On the way to the post office, she would rant and rave about what she really felt about him. It was a love/hate situation for her that tormented her constantly. I was scarred for life. Evidently, the world was not to be trusted, especially the people who were supposed to love and protect you the most.

It was a dysfunctional approach to relationships. If I wanted Mother to love me, it had better be *my* approach to those she despised, too. For a thirteen-year-old just beginning to establish a relationship with the real world, it was disastrous.

We were never allowed to use the word "alcoholic" to her. She said she wasn't an alcoholic. An unfeeling world and an insensitive family forced her drinking upon her. An alcoholic was a bum on the street. She just drank once in a while, so she could feel better about facing the world again. In fact, she said that she was a social drinker. I didn't dare tell her that there was nothing "social" about it. She didn't leave the house, when she was seriously drinking without stopping to eat or sleep.

Mother thought that if she went out with her much-younger friend, Judy, to a bar, then she was just having a few drinks to relax, to loosen up, to feel confident about herself in a social situation. That's why she drank. It was normal. She didn't want it mentioned again. There was absolutely nothing wrong with her behavior, in my mother's warped mind. It was the rest of the world that was cruel, insensitive, and judgmental. She was just doing what everyone else did. We didn't remind her that "everyone else" didn't use her living room carpet as a lavatory almost every Friday night.

When she was on a rampage, we ignored her running around the house, pulling out bottles of vodka from far back in drawers, deep in kitchen cabinets, rolled up in her hose, and we didn't ask her about the missing camera, my father's wristwatch, or the pearls he gave her one Christmas, that we knew she pawned for money to buy liquor.

"Don't you dare tell me what to do!"

"But Mother, you're going to hurt yourself."

"What do you care? You just expect me to wait on you hand and foot, like I had to do with my father."

She would start to sob uncontrollably when she mentioned her father. Now we had a morose mean drunk instead of an alcoholic, throwing things around to find her booze, screaming at us the whole while.

"He never loved me, you know. He didn't even like me."

My father would try to comfort her.

"Now, you know he really cared about you."

"Well, he sure had a strange way of showing it."

The sobbing had stopped. She was angry, again. She glared at my father and me, her eyes red-rimmed and bloodshot.

"What do you know about it? You're just as bad as he is. Always wanting something. Never giving me anything back."

I'd start to respond. My father would gesture for me to stay quiet with a finger against his mouth. He knew she wasn't really talking to us. Somewhere in her head, she was back with her father. He was making her feel miserable and unloved for the hundredth time.

Funny how she didn't realize she was doing the same to us. Alcoholics are self-centered and myopic. Drunks are selfish. Loved ones can be taken for granted. High functioning alcoholics like Mother, who could still hold down a job and maintain outside relationships, had to do "show and tell" for the rest of the world. But family must accept the bad with the good. As a kid, I didn't think that was a fair deal. But then,

I wasn't asked my opinion since I was a child. Interesting. I could hear and see the most awful things in my family and be treated more like a confidante than a kid, but when it came to criticizing what I thought was wrong, I was just a little girl, and didn't know what I was talking about.

We couldn't mention the tranquilizers or stimulants, either. Drug addicts were right next to the street drunks. That wasn't her, she said. She kept up the house, herself, her obligations as a wife and mother. She just needed something at the end of the day to relax her, to help her cope, to go back in where she was devalued and unloved. She was robbed of her childhood, so it was only natural to try to recapture it in bars, with too-young, drinking girlfriends, with drink after drink until she couldn't think a coherent thought. She wasn't to be held accountable; she wasn't to be blamed for what the world had done to her. Her own father had emotionally disowned her. If she slipped once in a while and drank a little too much to ease the remembered pain, well, who could say she was wrong?

So an alcoholic drug addict whose approval and love I was always seeking, primarily created my view of the world.

She taught me people will say one thing, but mean something else. Did I say enough, do enough, and show enough gratitude? Don't make friends; they'll betray you or leave you. Don't get attached to people or things. They're temporary. When you leave relationships, you cut them off completely. Leave before you get hurt. That was my way of dealing with the world when I lived with her, and when I didn't.

Mother had started as a beautiful, talented, sensitive, and loving girl. My father would show my sister and me photos of her when he first met her. He would tell us her fear of her father was strange to see, since when he was with her, she was strong, witty, and capable. When she was around her father, she was defensive, quiet, and withdrawn. The words "I'm sorry" and "You're right, Father" were usually all she would say.

When my father was with her away from her house, she was funny and eloquent. He hadn't known about her singing ability, until after they were married. I think he wanted us to know her for the fun-loving, charming, intelligent woman she really was.

When she was sleeping off a drunk upstairs, and my sister was sleeping, he would bring back memories of what she was like when he met her. He'd find the old photo album, and turn the pages full of photos of her when she was young.

"She laughed all the time when we were alone. I don't think I ever saw her laugh in her father's presence. This beautiful woman I knew to be smart, funny, and joyful, would stand across the room from her father with her head down, her shoulders slumped, and her voice in a whisper when she talked to him. And she only talked to him when he would speak directly to her, and tell her something."

"Why didn't she stand up to him?"

"Well, I think she was scared of him in a way. I guess she thought it would be worse for her and her stepmother, if she spoke back to him. Remember she saw what he was like when he was drinking. It must have terrified her."

"Why did she get married right away, and not go to music school?"

"I don't think she really believed her father was giving her a choice whether to go to a business school or a music college. She wanted to please him more than anything, so he would care about her. So she gave up her music, hoping he would compliment her on her decision. I don't think he ever did. Even when she was the top student they had. That was his way, how he had been taught to be when he was growing up."

He would look down at their wedding picture. My grandfather had wanted to save money on the wedding, so the minister married them in her back yard with a little cake and two witnesses. My father's parents had died. She wasn't asked if she wanted any of her girlfriends to be there. My father continued, "I think she loved me, but she also wanted to get out of that house as soon as she could. I was her only boyfriend that I know of. I wasn't making much money then, so her father disapproved of me, but she married me, anyway. Your mother is a very strong woman really. She did stand up to him about me. I never realized how hard that must have been for her. Alone in that house, her stepmother afraid to speak, her saying she was going to marry me. That took a lot of courage. I wish she could recognize how strong she is. We had some pretty lean times, but she stayed with me through it all, and even raised you girls without much money, and moving from place to place all the time when I was in the service. It was the best paying job around, but the military tells you what to do and where to go, and that's what you do. Your mother probably wanted a house with a white picket fence and a yard for her flowers. And maybe a church where she could sing and be appreciated for her voice."

He would close the album and sit quietly for a few minutes, thinking about those times. Somehow, even as young as I was and he had talked about adult things, I knew I should let him sit there without talking at him like I usually did. I was always grateful when he spent some time with me. I'd pester him to death, he would say, with all my questions.

Later, when I was older and had life experiences of my own, I would reflect back on those times with my father and the photo album, held together with old, faded-brown, velvet ribbon. I think he felt badly that he hadn't given her much of a life in the early years. That was probably the reason he tried to understand and sympathize with her, as she got further and further into her addictions. Maybe he thought he was the reason. She would say it often enough. But I don't think that was true. I think she truly loved him till the day he died. It was the alcohol and drugs that made her act out and say things she would never say, if she wasn't drugged up and drinking heavily. She was in constant emotional pain. In her day, the only way to deal with that was to drink and take tranquilizers.

He said it was her drinking that changed her. He felt he couldn't stop her. None of us could.

When I was growing up, she was still a pretty woman. She appeared to the outside world as a kind, considerate, and conscientious person who put others before herself. When I was with her and we'd meet anyone she worked with, she'd be that person. At home, she would say the worse things about them.

When she was drinking and she was raging, she would curse, throw things, and lose control of herself. She'd push away, if we tried to keep her from hurting herself. She'd scream and fight. Her face would be contorted with anger; she would scream-talk at us, and eventually fall to the floor in exhaustion. My father would take her upstairs. He'd come back down, and tell me she was sick and couldn't help herself. When she was herself, he'd say she was a wonderful mother and wife. It was her drinking and insecurities. It was confusing and terrifying for me. Mother didn't lose control when my sister was in the house. I think she wanted her to always think her mother was wonderful, kind, loving, and had no faults. But when my sister was out of the house at a sleepover or at a party, Mother felt free "to go on one of her tears."

My sister didn't escape, though. When my father died, Mother came to live with her. She became her caretaker. Fortunately for Mother, my sister has always been emotionally self-sufficient. There are no grounds for bitterness or remorse. Unlike me, she didn't hold grudges or become vulnerable to others' perceived opinions. Mother never set her up to be torn down.

I have not seen Mother in years. Perhaps it is time, before it is too late for both of us. Hopefully, I am not as needy and dependent upon the way the world envisioned me, so that when I was in my skinny cycle, I became what I feared the most – Mother.

Not a Nice Person

My way of life when I was slender and people were attracted to me, included making denigrating comments about myself, refusing to accept compliments, putting others before myself, and clutching at anyone who showed they liked me.
I remember saying to those who befriended me that I would die for them.

But if I felt someone had hurt me, I was the bitterest enemy. Since I was personable and intelligent, people would be drawn to me. If they wanted to remain in my circle, they had to adopt my point of view about anyone.

I had a scathing wit. Words and actions were fierce weapons. I was a natural leader, so it was easy to isolate the person I disliked from others. If you wanted to remain in my group, you had better follow my lead. I could keep it up for months.

Other than my aberrant personality traits, I also had my perfectionism and obsessive-compulsive behavior to deal with. Perfect papers, everything in its place, clothes and shoes lined up, nothing askew was the norm for me. I had to stop myself from straightening pictures, putting objects from smallest to biggest, correcting grammar when people spoke, fixing their clothes while they were wearing them. Irritation and impatience with others were common. Dismissing people and things because of perceived imperfections was a daily occurrence. When I was thin and admired, if something was broken or someone was imperfect around me, I threw them aside and never looked back.

Since my father was in the Air Force and we moved every two to four years, I did not allow myself to get attached to people or places. I found it amusing when I had been best friends with a girl for several years, I went over to her house to say goodbye, and she had already replaced me. Her mother answered my knock.

"Is Kathy home?"

Her mother looked pityingly at me, and tried to shut the door a bit, as she prepared to say something. I heard laughter and looked past her. There on the stairs I had run up so many times, when Kathy and I would race to her room after school, to discuss the day's events, especially the girls we hated that particular week and the boys we loved, was my friend-for-life Kathy and her new best friend. I smiled, turned around and walked away. I didn't hear the sympathetic words Kathy's mother would have tried to say. It didn't matter, anyway. I didn't resent Kathy for replacing me. That was how life was. And that was how I treated anyone who was my temporary best friend in the future. As my mother would say, "Live and learn." Life was hard, and then you die.

When I got fat, I was the biggest imperfection in my world. I would fix it. Just like lining up my toothbrush and toothpaste, I lined up my bottles of phentermine, made my bulimic schedules, and listened only to the voice that told me I was worthless until I lost weight. It was the sole voice that counted.

I had let myself get out of control. How had I let that happen? I had planned and executed things perfectly all my life. What had I missed? Low self-esteem and fear of being unloved, had led to a frenzy of emotional eating. I knew what I had to do. Appearance is everything. I had learned that from Mother. The world agreed. I had the addictive tools to alter my brain and repair my unloved body. And of course, I did everything to perfection. It would only be a matter of time.

End Note

Fifteen years is a long time to do anything. Doing something as destructive as bulimia and amphetamines, will eventually catch up with you. It caught up with me at what was supposed to be one of the best times of my life.

I didn't pay attention to the wakeup calls my body was giving me. I was doing it damage. It was screaming back at me. I chose not to listen. That deluded fat-girl point of view again.

Irreparable and *inevitable* are two words I didn't think would apply to me in my twenties. I had all kinds of things going wrong. I didn't do anything about them. I had to be loved. I had to be thin

Whatever it took-- diet pills, shots, throwing up fifteen times a day, I would be thin if it killed me. It looks like it would, after all

Coda

I'm in my thin state now. The anti-depressant I take is one of the most potent they make. I take the highest dosage. It keeps the addictions at bay. They're always there, though – waiting. I won't outlive them.

www.ingramcontent.com/pod-product-compliance
Lightning Source LLC
Chambersburg PA
CBHW032059280526
45784CB00012B/162